T0178317

Success in Academic Surgery

Series editors
Lillian Kao, University of Texas Health Science Center at Houston, Houston, Texas, USA
Herbert Chen, University of Wisconsin, Madison, Wisconsin, USA

More information about this series at http://www.springer.com/series/11216

Michael J. Englesbe • Michael O. Meyers
Editors

A How To Guide For Medical Students

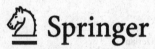

Editors
Michael J. Englesbe
Transplantation Surgery
University of Michigan Health Systems
Ann Arbour, MI, USA

Michael O. Meyers
Surgical Oncology
University of North Carolina School
   of Medicine
Chapel Hill, NC, USA

ISSN 2194-7481   ISSN 2194-749X   (electronic)
Success in Academic Surgery
ISBN 978-3-319-42895-6   ISBN 978-3-319-42897-0   (eBook)
DOI 10.1007/978-3-319-42897-0

Library of Congress Control Number: 2016958314

Printed on acid-free paper

This Springer imprint is published by Springer Nature
The registered company is Springer International Publishing AG Switzerland

Foreword

This book is designed to help medical students who have an interest in a surgical career prepare to successfully pursue the residency of their choice. While some of the content focuses on academic surgery, much of the information will be of use to all students interested in surgery even if their career goals do not include an academic career. Regardless of what point a student is in their medical training, this book should provide useful information and guidance.

Surgical Oncology   Michael O. Meyers
University of North Carolina School of Medicine
Chapel Hill, NC, USA
Transplantation Surgery   Michael J. Englesbe
University of Michigan Health Systems
Ann Arbour, MI, USA

Contents

Contributors

Anthony Charles University of North Carolina, Chapel Hill, NC, USA

Karole T. Collier University of Pennsylvania, Philadelphia, PA, USA

Shannon L. Cramm University of Michigan, Ann Arbor, MI, USA
Johns Hopkins School of Medicine, Baltimore, MD, USA

David Cron University of Michigan, Ann Arbor, MI, USA

Jason Crowner University of North Carolina, Chapel Hill, NC, USA

Stephanie DeBolle University of Michigan, Ann Arbor, MI, USA

Keith Delman Emory University School of Medicine, Atlanta, GA, USA

Scott C. DeRoo Columbia University, New York, NY, USA

Michael J. Englesbe Transplantation Surgery, University of Michigan Health Systems, Ann Arbor, MI, USA

Jared R. Gallaher University of North Carolina, Chapel Hill, NC, USA

Amir A. Ghaferi Department of Surgery, University of Michigan, Ann Arbor, MI, USA

Jason P. Glotzbach Assistant Professor, Division of Cardiothoracic Surgery, University of Utah, Salt Lake City, UT, USA

Jacob A. Greenberg University of Wisconsin, Madison, WI, USA

David T. Hughes University of Michigan, Ann Arbor, MI, USA

C. Scott Hultman University of North Carolina, Chapel Hill, NC, USA

Charles Hwang University of Michigan, Ann Arbor, MI, USA

Hee Soo Jung University of Wisconsin, Madison, WI, USA

Rachel R. Kelz University of Pennsylvania, Philadelphia, PA, USA

Sanjay Krishnaswami Oregon Health Science University, Portland, OR, USA

Michael T. LeCompte Vanderbilt University Medical Center, Nashville, TN, USA

Scott A. LeMaire Michael E. DeBakey Department of Surgery, Baylor College of Medicine, Houston, TX, USA

Benjamin Levi University of Michigan, Ann Arbor, MI, USA

Alyssa Mazurek University of Michigan, Ann Arbor, MI, USA

Katharine L. McGinigle University of North Carolina, Chapel Hill, NC, USA

Michael O. Meyers Surgical Oncology, University of North Carolina School of Medicine, Chapel Hill, NC, USA

Jason Pradarelli Brigham and Women's Hospital, Boston, MA, USA

Carla M. Pugh University of Wisconsin, Madison, WI, USA

Laura N. Purcell University of North Carolina, Chapel Hill, NC, USA

Rishindra M. Reddy University of Michigan, Ann Arbor, MI, USA

Michelle Roughton University of North Carolina, Chapel Hill, NC, USA

George A. Sarosi Jr. University of Florida, Gainesville, FL, USA

Dorry Segev Johns Hopkins School of Medicine, Baltimore, MD, USA

Christiana Shaw University of Florida, Gainesville, FL, USA

Jahnavi Srinivasan Emory University School of Medicine, Atlanta, GA, USA

Melissa K. Stewart Vanderbilt University Medical Center, Nashville, TN, USA

Mamta Swaroop Northwestern Feinberg School of Medicine, Chicago, IL, USA

Kyla P. Terhune Vanderbilt University Medical Center, Nashville, TN, USA

Patrick Underwood University of Florida, Gainesville, FL, USA

Part I
Clinical Training and Making Sure Surgery Is Right for You

Chapter 1
Why Consider a Career in Academic Surgery

Michael O. Meyers

Abstract This chapter gives perspective on a career in academic surgery and some of the reasons a student would consider such a career. Surgery itself has many rewards, regardless of the setting in which one practices. The privilege of taking care of patients, the trust people have in allowing us to operate on them and the close bonds we form with patients and their families are some of the intangible rewards to a surgical career. We really do make a difference in people's lives. While this chapter is focused on why one might consider a career in academic surgery, I would hope that much of it is relevant to anyone considering a surgical career.

1.1 Introduction

This chapter gives perspective on a career in academic surgery and some of the reasons a student would consider such a career. Surgery itself has many rewards, regardless of the setting in which one practices. The privilege of taking care of patients, the trust people have in allowing us to operate on them and the close bonds we form with patients and their families are some of the intangible rewards to a surgical career. We really do make a difference in people's lives. While this chapter is focused on why one might consider a career in academic surgery, I would hope that much of it is relevant to anyone considering a surgical career.

As I began to write this chapter, I found myself taking inventory of my own career path and the key choices that led me both to academic surgery and the route I have taken since I finished my training. I wish I could say it was a series of 5-year plans and everything proceeded in a premeditated and orderly fashion. That would be a much tidier picture. But the reality is that if you had asked me when I completed my training where I would be in 10 years, the picture I would have painted would bear only a small resemblance to what my career has looked like. I don't say that to discount the concept of setting thoughtful goals and putting down on paper, with the help of mentors, those things you hope to accomplish both short-term and long-term. That is a critical and necessary step on the pathway to success and

M.O. Meyers, MD (✉)
Surgical Oncology, University of North Carolina School of Medicine, Chapel Hill, NC, USA
e-mail: michael_meyers@med.unc.edu

© Springer International Publishing Switzerland 2017
M.J. Englesbe, M.O. Meyers (eds.), *A How To Guide For Medical Students,*
Success in Academic Surgery, DOI 10.1007/978-3-319-42897-0_1

something I would encourage everyone to do. But I am suggesting that the path isn't always a straight line and you should look for opportunitis as they arise that may deviate your course in a positive way. When I chose to enter surgery as a medical student, my primary goal was to become a good surgeon. I didn't have the foresight to think about what setting I might practice in or the ambition to think I could or would end up as an academic surgeon. While not true of many in academic surgery, I'm sure I am not alone. As I considered this, I thought this was the perfect way to begin explaining my thoughts on why one should consider a career in academic surgery. I have had the opportunity to be: a busy surgeon who as a surgical oncologist has the privilege of literally operating on the skin and it's contents; a scientific investigator in clinical trials; a collaborator in translational and health services research; a teacher of medical students and surgical residents (the latter one of the greatest sources of ongoing enjoyment in my career); a leader as the program director of a surgical residency program (a job I couldn't have even defined at the time I completed my training); a mentor to students, residents and junior faculty. While some of these are things I actively pursued from the beginning and would have predicted, many others are not. What other type of surgical career can give you such broad experience and opportunity? In academic surgery, there is never a boring or rote day where you get up in the morning and dread the sameness of your work. You might not look forward to every day, just as in most jobs or professions there are things you enjoy more than others. But there is never the dread of mindless sameness to this career. The following paragraphs give my top reasons why you should choose an academic surgical career, many of which will be fleshed out further in the ensuing chapters.

1.2   Broad Career Opportunities

A career as an academic surgeon can follow many pathways. The historical model of the 'triple threat' surgeon who was a master teacher, a busy and expert clinician and someone who furthered their field scientifically through basic science research is by no means the only pathway to a surgical career (Stein 2013). While this paradigm still exists and does play a critical role in academic surgery, there are a number of ways in which a surgical career can lead to academic success. Greater recognition is now given to the many roles that are necessary to make departments of surgery successful and opportunities exist for clinical, educational, administrative and broad-based research efforts. Departments of surgery have collectively become the 'triple threat' by fostering an environment where every faculty member contributes to the clinical, research and education missions, but not necessarily all three of these (Staveley-O'Carroll et al. 2005). However, by working as a group and complimenting each other, excellence can be achieved collectively in all missions and faculty members can identify their own contribution to something bigger than any one individual. Busy clinicians who develop and build clinical programs not only contribute to the financial success of surgery departments and the education mission by training residents and fellows, but are often engaged in clinical trials, translational research partnerships, investigation of new technology and other research endeavors. Research careers can take on many looks. Basic and translational research remains an important part of surgical investigation and despite recognized challenges can be a pathway to success in surgical research (Smythe 2010; Kibbe et al. 2015). But scientific investigation and funding in surgical careers involving health services and outcomes research, global health, quality of care and education have also become viable career choices. The growth in health services research in the last 15 years has been exponential. Similarly, global surgery has been recognized in the recent past as an important mission from all perspectives including clinical care and program building, training and research and is the foundation for an increasing number of academic surgical careers (Zerhouni et al. 2015; Taro et al. 2016). Education remains an important part of the academic surgical career, but this too has evolved. While clinical teaching remains important and is part of the career of nearly every academic surgeon, there is recognition that expert educators are a necessary and important part of the successful academic enterprise. This is covered in detail in the subsequent chapter on surgical education, but this too can have many avenues for developing expertise and opportunities for success with regard to program development, administration and research. Finally, the practice setting for an academic surgeon is now recognized as much more broad than it used to be. Not only is 'academic surgery' practiced at university-based hospitals, but much more broadly in traditionally 'private' hospitals. These institutions conduct clinical research, train residents and provide excellent clinical care. While the research engines may not be as well developed in some of these settings, there are broad opportunities for surgeons to fulfill the goals of an academic practice.

1.3   Personal Fulfillment and Being Part of Something Bigger

The sense of accomplishment that a surgeon has with their job is not unique to academic practice. The privilege of operating on patients and making them better is shared across the discipline. But in an academic practice this often entails taking care of the most advanced diseases and working as a team. The relationships that you develop with not just patients but your entire professional working group can be very rewarding. These close relationships contribute to job satisfaction. Surgeons in this setting often have the opportunity to be leaders of their teams, which also contributes to a sense of personal fulfillment. The academic surgeon also has the opportunity to teach and mentor both medical students and surgical residents. The personal reward of acting not just as a teacher but a mentor is difficult to measure objectively, but plays a large role in why many people are committed to an academic surgical career even if they are not involved in funded research efforts. Finally, the sense of being part of a team is a very satisfying part of being an academic surgeon. Accomplishments of the group beyond ones own personal success contributes to the sense of being part of something bigger than yourself and is itself rewarding.

This is true in your clinical teams and also in watching surgical trainees grow and mature. For me, one of my favorite days every year is the annual resident graduation celebration in our surgery department. There are few things I do professionally that are as rewarding as seeing surgical residents progress from interns to graduating residents.

1.4 Innovation and Intellectual Stimulation

An exciting part of being an academic surgeon is the chance to be constantly stimulated intellectually. At some point in every surgical career, the operations you do and the clinical care will become routine. While everyone evolves over their career and learns new things, as an academic surgeon you will be constantly challenged by your peers, your trainees and your collaborators. This may be to learn new techniques or apply new technology in the operating room, often pushed by your trainees. It may be to consider scientific questions and be part of finding a solution. It may be your own interest in answering a research question. This is true both in the operating and outside the operating room where you have the opportunity to work with collaborators across many disciplines and learn new things. The adage attributed to Louis Pasteur, "chance favors the prepared mind", applies to academic surgery where there are many opportunities for people who are interested and open to new things.

1.5 It's Fun!

The final aspect of an academic surgical career that I would highlight is that it's fun. You are able to work with like-minded people who are smart and interesting. Someone is always asking a new question or thinking about things in a way that you hadn't considered. There is a constant infusion of new and bright minds in your daily world with new students and residents arriving at regular intervals, many of whom challenge you to be smarter and better than you would be if they weren't around. Not every aspect of every day is painted with joy to be sure and there are days that present significant challenges. But I can honestly say that every day, some aspect of my job is fun and interesting.

1.6 Why Not Be an Academic Surgeon

It seems only fair that after spending several paragraphs writing about why you should consider a career in academic surgery, that I spend a little time on why you might not want to consider this path. For starters, money should not be a primary motivation if you desire an academic surgical career. By no means has anyone taken a vow of poverty regardless of what surgical specialty they practice or what setting they practice in. But in general compensation has traditonally been better in non-academic settings where the focus is primarily on clinical care and at least in our current system of compensation, volume of patient care. While this is slowly changing, it is likely there will always be a difference. Most university hospitals are not the model of efficiency either (although as a whole this is improving), which can lead to its own set of frustrations. In general, if your primary motivation is to build a busy practice and work in as efficient a system as possible, while spending little time on anything else, then a job in academic surgery probably isn't the right thing for you. That doesn't mean surgery isn't the right choice as there are still many rewarding aspects of surgery in a non-academic setting. But you should consider carefully the motivation for your career and shape your choice of practice accordingly.

1.7 Summary

In summary, I would suggest never has there been a better time to consider becoming an academic surgeon. The number of opportunities to make your own career path and be successful are innumerable. A career in academic surgery can be fulfilling both professionally and personally and will continually challenge you to be better as a physician, a teacher, a leader and as a person. In a treatise on academic medical centers published in 1999 titled 'Understanding Academic Medical Centers', Joe Simone, a former director of St. Jude Children's Research Hospital and the Huntsman Cancer Institute at the University of Utah, highlighted many of the challenges and the joys of the academic medical center. Part of his conclusion read: "We have the privilege of working in a profession that helps the sick and dying while we are engaged in intellectual inquiry. Our profession is still highly respected by society, and we are paid quite well for doing something most of us love to do." This is still true some 15 years later I can think of no better words to summarize why you should consider a career in academic surgery.

The following chapters are designed to help you consider in more detail a career in academic surgery. We have tried to provide an overview of what an academic surgical career can look like from the perspective of several people who have chosen disparate career paths and are accomplished in their fields. There are perspectives on wellness and surgery as well as thoughts from a residency program director on the qualities that yield success in surgical trainees. Several chapters are devoted to how to prepare yourself as a student to successfully pursue surgery residency and begin setting yourself up for a career. Finally, we the review the match process, how to think about choosing a residency program and some advice from current residents about things they recommend paying attention to as a student. Hopefully this book can provide some guidance to you in pursuing your career goals in surgery.

References

Kibbe MR, Dardik A, Velazquez OC, Conte MS. The vascular surgeon-scientist: a 15-year report of the Society for Vascular Surgery Foundation/National Heart, Lung, and Blood Institute-mentored Career Development Award Program. J Vasc Surg. 2015;61(4):1050–7.

Smythe WR. The future of academic surgery. Acad Med. 2010;85(5):768–74.

Staveley-O'Carroll K, Pan M, Meier A, Han D, McFadden D, Souba W. Developing the young academic surgeon. J Surg Res. 2005;128(2):238–42.

Stein SL. Scholarship in academic surgery: history, challenges, and ideas for the future. Clin Colon Rectal Surg. 2013;26(4):207–11.

Taro T, Yao C, Ly S, Wipfli H, Magee K, Vanderburg R, Magee 3rd W. The global surgery partnership: an innovative partnership for education, research, and service. Acad Med. 2016;91(1):75–8.

Zerhouni YA, Abu-Bonsrah N, Mehes M, Goldstein S, Buyske J, Abdullah F. General surgery education: a systematic review of training worldwide. Lancet. 2015;385 Suppl 2:S39.

Chapter 2
What Does an Academic Career Look Like in Surgical Education?

Hee Soo Jung and Carla M. Pugh

Abstract Surgical education is rapidly growing as a formal career option. Choosing a focus area is the key to success. Opportunities exist at the medical student, resident, fellow, and practicing physician level. There is also the option of focusing on teaching, curriculum development and evaluation, or traditional experimental or investigational research. This chapter will focus on the various career opportunities in surgical education and provide examples of real-life career paths demonstrating the many options for a successful, fulfilling academic career in surgical education.

2.1 Introduction

Hee Soo Jung and Carla M. Pugh

Surgical education is rapidly growing as a formal career option with the opportunity for both local and national recognition Pugh and Sippel (2013). Choosing a focus area is the key to success. For some, the primary interest is medical student education. Others may choose to focus on residents or fellows while others show a strong interest in continuing medical education. For each of these areas, there is also the option of choosing to focus on teaching, curriculum development and evaluation, or traditional experimental or investigational research. This chapter will review the various career opportunities in surgical education and provide examples of real-life career paths demonstrating the many options for a successful, fulfilling career in surgical education. In addition, we highlight ways that a medical student might be able to get involved in surgical education as a student, an endeavor that can lead to the identification of mentors who can be influential in finding the right residency program.

H.S. Jung, MD • C.M. Pugh, MD, PhD (✉)
University of Wisconsin, Madison, WI, USA
e-mail: jung@surgery.wisc.edu; pugh@surgery.wisc.edu

© Springer International Publishing Switzerland 2017
M.J. Englesbe, M.O. Meyers (eds.), *A How To Guide For Medical Students,*
Success in Academic Surgery, DOI 10.1007/978-3-319-42897-0_2

2.2   Choosing Your Area of Focus

What are you most passionate about? Do you find yourself going home each day from a busy clinical practice wondering if the medical students really understand a disease process, operation or treatment regimen? Or, do you believe you can shorten the learning curve for residents and fellows? If you aren't sure where to start there are a number of options; (a) Conduct a personal inventory. This will provide a structured way of reflecting on those specific, personal experiences that sparked your interest; (b) Discuss your interests with your mentors, chairman and other department leaders as they may have insight on areas of local and national importance; (c) Partner with like-minded colleagues. For example, you may want to visit your local simulation center and find out if there are other faculty already developing curricula or conducting research in your area of interest. The benefit of this approach is partnering with someone that may already have dedicated infrastructure or personnel.

Focus on Medical Students The most common leadership position, for those who want a career relating to medical student education, is the Clerkship Director. As a student, you will know this person as they will likely be your primary point of faculty contact during your surgery clerkship. This person usually works closely with a Clerkship Coordinator to facilitate all aspects of medical student education relating to the department of surgery. This is a very rewarding and usually well supported role in the department and the medical school. There are numerous opportunities to conduct research in this role if there is an interest and your clerkship director may be a great point of contact as a student to begin to be involved in research, particularly those focused on surgical education. This person may also have appointments in the medical school relating to curriculum oversight and reform.

Focus on Residents and Fellows The most common leadership position, for those who want a career relating to education of residents and fellows, is the Program or Fellowship Director. This person usually works closely with a Program Administrator to facilitate all aspects of graduate medical education (residents and fellows). This is also a very rewarding and usually well supported role in the department and the medical school. These individuals are another great point of contact as a student and may be helpful early in your medical career in giving guidance and mentorship with regard to a potential career focused on surgical education. There are numerous opportunities to conduct research in this role as well. This person works with medical school leaders, usually a Designated Institutional Official (DIO), to help maintain ACGME accreditation.

Focus on Continuing Medical Education Over the past few years there has been an increase in the amount of attention being paid to continuing medical education (CME) as an area for research and leadership Sachdeva (2005). While there is still a paucity of formal leadership positions in this area in surgical departments, most academic medical centers have an Office of Continuing Professional

Development that may serve as the support for persons interested in working in this area. Under the umbrella of the American Board of Medical Specialties, the specialty boards have had an increased focus on developing and restructuring their Maintenance of Certification (MOC) programs. As a result, unique partnerships between Quality Improvement divisions in the hospital and CME in the medical school are on the rise in academic medical centers. These new partnerships present fertile ground for leadership positions and education research.

2.3 Research in Surgical Education

The number of research papers written in surgical education has been on a steep rise since the early 2000s. The influx of research methods from mainstream education research to the surgical profession has had a tremendous impact on the science of surgical education. In addition, the recent push for explicit documentation of learning and competency has provided a sound foundation for scientific exploration, validation, and experimentation with a wide variety of surveys, checklists and other performance tools. Moreover, the vast development and utilization of simulation centers in today's medical centers has allowed researchers and trainees to convene in a controlled and reproducible environment that further supports the research enterprise. From curriculum development and evaluation to the use of advanced performance measurement technologies such as sensors and motion tracking, research in surgical education covers a wide variety of topics and engenders numerous cross-disciplinary collaborations with fellow researchers in a number of disciplines including education, engineering, cognitive psychology and many more.

2.4 The Career Path

The first step in developing a career in surgical education is deciding what path to take. In addition to the formal department based leadership positions in surgical education, faculty can take numerous paths in teaching and research. During your residency, you will also have a number of opportunities to be involved in surgical education. You will certainly be a teacher of students and other learners. But you will also have the opportunity to begin laying the foundation for an academic career by being involved in education based research or formal teaching education.

Faculty committed to excellence in teaching have a special relationship with students, residents and fellows. This relationship provides an incredible honor and a fulfilling opportunity for faculty who pursue this as their primary path in surgical education. In addition to lectures and time in the simulation lab, these faculty carve out a significant amount of time providing feedback in various clinical venues often yielding praise and teaching awards from the trainees.

Faculty with advanced or specialized operative skills can take the path of developing CME level courses that achieve national and local recognition and serve as a venue for training practicing clinicians who wish to learn a new procedure, technique or instrument. Faculty with an interest in licensing, policy and standard setting may seek to become involved with the American Board of Surgery or the ACGME. These opportunities are highly coveted and usually require a certain level of professional success prior to appointment.

Lastly, promotion and tenure guidelines provide valuable information on how to get promoted based on surgical education. Curriculum development, teaching and leadership roles, and the more traditional grant funding and journal publications are all included in the promotion packet of surgical educators.

The research path, which is not mutually exclusive from the leadership and teaching paths, can take on many forms. Faculty who pursue and obtain NIH or DOD level funding for their research in surgical education share their clinical time with running a research lab. The composition of the research lab depends on the research focus. Education, engineering and other disciplines are increasingly collaborating with surgeons to conduct innovative research in educational technology development and performance measurement. Technology based laboratories in surgical education focus on developing and evaluating educational technologies including hardware and software – virtual reality, anatomical models and virtual patients are a few examples. Performance based laboratories spend more time focused on the metrics of performance including measuring learning curves, psychomotor and cognitive skills. As one can imagine, the mix of personnel in a technology based lab might look very different than a performance measurement laboratory.

While there are different levels of funding that can be achieved by surgical education faculty, being a productive, well-known researcher does not require high level funding. A strong commitment to teaching, learning, assessment and excellence is all that is required. Faculty with a passion for surgical training will find a way to combine their clinical practice with the research they wish to accomplish.

2.5   Special Considerations

Advanced Degrees Though obtaining an advanced degree is not a requirement, it does afford the opportunity to learn a set of skills and educational theories that may be difficult master otherwise. Master's degree programs in medical education as well as traditional education are both viable options. Things to consider when choosing one versus the other include: curricular focus, scheduling flexibility (i.e. online or night courses) and access to surgical mentors to compliment the degree mentors. Surgical mentorship during this time is extremely important as it is uncommon for faculty in the school of education to know which societies you should join, which journals you should publish in and which meetings you should attend. A doctoral degree is a longer commitment. However, it may be worth the effort if you have a strong interest in the conduct of educational research using a wide variety of qualitative and quantitative methods. In addition, statistics show that physicians with doctoral level degrees are more likely to obtain higher level NIH or DOD funding. A strong mentoring team and a clear vision of what you would like to accomplish in your career will help you make the right decision for you.

National Meetings The Association for Surgical Education (ASE) and the Association of Program Directors in Surgery (APDS) host an annual meeting entitled "Surgical Education Week" (https://surgicaleducation.com/annual-meeting-information). This joint meeting is the largest and longest standing meeting focused on surgical education. This meeting is a great place for students to potentially present surgical education-based research and develop an even broader perspective on the world of surgical education in general and surgical education research. Becoming involved in some of these efforts with surgical mentors early on in your medical school career will afford you greatest opportunity to participate in research that can lead to your being able to attend and present your own work at these meetings. In addition, the Academic Surgical Congress (a joint meeting of the Association of Academic Surgery and Society of University Surgeons) and the American College of Surgeons Annual Clinical Congress meetings both have surgical education tracks for sharing education research. All of these venues provide excellent opportunities for mentorship in surgical education as well as collaboration.

Publishing Your Work Publishing is critical for an academic career in surgery. While there are no journal restrictions relating to well-written education research papers with an excellent protocol and research methods, there are a few journals that have a higher percentage and interest in education research. If you have a strong desire to have an academic surgical career focused on education, begin working on research efforts that can be published early in your medical school career. The official journal for the ASE is the American Journal of Surgery. The official journal for the APDS is the Journal of Surgical Education. The official journal for the AAS is the Journal of Surgical Research and the official journal of the SUS is the Journal of Surgery. Journals that are not specific to surgical education include Academic Medicine and Simulation in Healthcare. Both of these journals, as well as many of specialty journals, may publish research relating to surgical education.

2.6 How to Get Involved as a Student

Start as soon as you identify an interest in surgery and think you might have a desire to pursue surgical education as a meaningful part of your career. Consider the above areas of educational expertise and think about which of these might fit best with your interests. It is likely that someone in your medical school or surgery department is working on all of the above-mentioned areas as they are critical to the function of your department. There are many opportunities for you to become engaged in some aspect of your department's surgical education efforts. Most people won't say no to a volunteer who is willing to put in the work. This might begin with something as simple as helping set up simulation labs but may grow into a research project in that same simulation lab. The clerkship director, residency program director or simulation lab director are all great places to start as they will be connected broadly and can give you guidance. In addition to starting early, look for opportunities to be involved in research projects that can lead to presentation and publications. Your mentors will help guide you, but these are things that will help distinguish you from other applicants to surgery programs and afford you opportunities to attend meetings that will help you gain knowledge and grow.

2.7 Summary

An academic career in surgical education can take a variety of paths. Beginning your involvement as a student can help set you up for success during residency and in your career. Choosing a specific area of interest and finding a mentor are key first steps and this can begin as a student. Obtaining funding, publishing your work and presenting at national meetings are additional, important steps to achieving a successful career in surgical education and can begin early in your career as well. Teaching awards, leadership positions and honorific appointments at a national level are all in reach with a strategic plan for success.

References

Aggarwal R, Korndorffer J, Cannon-Bowers J, eds. ACS principles and practice for simulation and surgical education research. 2014. https://www.facs.org/education/accreditation/aei/resources/research-manual#sthash.cz5tBiHu.dpuf.

Pugh CM, Sippel RS, editors. Success in academic surgery: developing a career in surgical education. London: Springer; 2013.

Sachdeva AK. Acquiring skills in new procedures and technology: the challenge and the opportunity. Arch Surg. 2005;140(4):387–9.

Chapter 3
Basic and Translational Science in a Surgical Career

Scott A. LeMaire

Abstract Basic and translational science—in which investigators perform laboratory experiments to answer fundamental biological questions and directly link laboratory discoveries to clinical care—is essential to expanding our understanding of surgical disease and improving our ability to care for affected patients. Academic surgeons play a crucial role in surgical basic science because of their expertise in the clinical manifestations of disease, the nuances of operative treatment, and the challenges of postoperative care. This expertise imparts the surgeon with a unique perspective that informs clinically relevant basic science hypotheses. As the gap between clinical care and fundamental science continues to expand, the surgeon-scientist who speaks both languages is ideally suited to ensure that basic research focuses on clinically-relevant questions and that important new discoveries are ultimately translated into improvements in patient care.

Basic and translational science—in which investigators perform laboratory experiments to answer fundamental biological questions and directly link laboratory discoveries to clinical care—is essential to expanding our understanding of surgical disease and improving our ability to care for affected patients. Academic surgeons play a crucial role in surgical basic science because of their expertise in the clinical manifestations of disease, the nuances of operative treatment, and the challenges of postoperative care. This expertise imparts the surgeon with a unique perspective that informs clinically relevant basic science hypotheses. The critical role of the surgeon in conducting basic science was wonderfully articulated by Dr. Francis D. Moore, the esteemed surgeon-scientist who served as Surgeon-in-Chief at Harvard Medical School's Peter Bent Brigham Hospital for nearly three decades (1948–1976) and led

S.A. LeMaire (✉)
Michael E. DeBakey Department of Surgery, Baylor College of Medicine, Houston, TX, USA
e-mail: slemarie@bcm.com

© Springer International Publishing Switzerland 2017
M.J. Englesbe, M.O. Meyers (eds.), *A How To Guide For Medical Students*,
Success in Academic Surgery, DOI 10.1007/978-3-319-42897-0_3

pioneering research in organ transplantation and the metabolic response to surgery (Moore 1958; Folkman 2006; Hill 2006).

> In undertaking a year in fundamental research, learning how to use the new methods of nuclear physics for the study of surgical illness, I was crossing a bridge from the bedside to the laboratory, from the operating room to the world of basic science. In any medical field it is important for some clinicians to cross this bridge and bring back to the bedside whatever they can find out there (Moore 1995).

Dr. Moore's description of surgeon-scientists as "bridge-tenders" is perhaps even more relevant today in the era of incredibly complex molecular biology and rapidly advancing technology. As the gap between clinical care and fundamental science continues to expand, the surgeon-scientist who speaks both languages is ideally suited to ensure that basic research focuses on clinically-relevant questions and that important new discoveries are ultimately translated into improvements in patient care (LeMaire 2012).

Although the bridge-tender paradigm continues to apply to surgeon scientists, the nature of this process has markedly changed during the past few decades. In the past, when surgical science focused primarily on pathophysiology and the development of new operative treatments, it was common for clinicians to independently lead groundbreaking laboratory research projects. As the focus shifted to increasingly complex molecular biology, many surgeons partnered with non-clinician PhD scientists who had the expertise necessary to apply cutting-edge approaches to understanding the molecular basis of disease and its treatment. Today, surgeons commonly work with multidisciplinary teams of scientists to tackle challenging problems in basic research.

The participation of surgeons in integrated basic science research teams is both essential and highly rewarding (Economou 2016). Dr. James Economou recently emphasized the expanding importance of the "team science" approach to solving the world's most pressing research questions.

> The major biomedical research themes that will command our attention in the 21st century—neuroscience, cardiovascular disease, oncology—will require large team science efforts integrating a diversity of scientific disciplines, including biology, engineering, sociology, chemistry, and medicine. These scientific teams must also integrate diversity in gender, race, and ethnicity to enrich and add value to their discoveries and to better serve a diverse and multicultural society (Economou 2014).

Direct involvement of surgeons in team science is paramount because of their firsthand insight into the clinical aspects of disease and treatment. The opportunity to work with experts in highly diverse fields—such as molecular physiology, cell biology, biomedical engineering, genomics, proteomics, metabolomics, bioinformatics, nanobiotechnology, and drug discovery—toward solving complex scientific problems relevant to surgical patients broadens the surgeon's knowledge base and perspective. Furthermore, because surgeons lead similarly diverse teams when operating and providing perioperative care to patients on a daily basis, surgeons are often very well-suited to navigate the challenges of leading multidisciplinary research teams as well (Bennett et al. 2010; National Research Council 2015).

Team science also expands opportunities for obtaining funding because many funding agencies, including the National Institutes of Health and the National Science Foundation, have become increasingly committed to promoting multidisciplinary research.

There are many ways to gain exposure to laboratory research during medical school. For students who are already committed to developing a career that will include basic science research, several medical schools offer medical scientist training programs that confer both MD and PhD degrees, as well as shorter research tracks that enable students to spend one full year working with a faculty mentor in the laboratory. Students who are unable to enroll in one of these formal programs or are merely curious about laboratory research at their current stage should be encouraged to seek other opportunities to work in a lab. Because participating in basic science projects during medical school can be more challenging than participating in clinical and educational research projects—which generally lend themselves to off-hours work while students are engrossed in demanding preclinical classes and clinical rotations—many students who are interested in learning about or conducting basic science will spend dedicated time in a lab during the summer or a formal research elective. Regardless of the format of the laboratory experience, it is important to select an appropriate mentor (see Chap. 8: Developing a research portfolio as a medical student).

Students and residents often ask whether it is important to work in a laboratory that focuses on their presumed surgical specialty. When possible, being mentored by a surgeon-scientist in one's area of interest can be beneficial for a few reasons. Perhaps most importantly, the mentor in this situation can serve as an excellent role model by demonstrating how a surgeon can successfully balance clinical and academic responsibilities. In addition, it is never too early to begin gaining expertise in a specific field or to begin building a network of colleagues by meeting others in the field, many of whom may be able to provide future support during the residency application process and beyond. Having said this, it is fairly uncommon and certainly not necessary for a student to work in a lab focused on their future subspecialty. Students may not be able to find a suitable laboratory in their area of interest or may not yet know what specialty they intend to pursue. In these common situations, students can take comfort in knowing that the overall quality of the educational experience and the personal "fit" of a given mentor and their lab are far more important factors to consider when choosing a mentor. Regardless of the specific area of focus, a high quality educational experience in a lab will enable the student to learn fundamental research skills, such as developing and testing a hypothesis; designing rigorous experiments that include proper controls; critically analyzing data with appropriate statistical tests; and presenting and publishing scientific work. All of these skills will become part of a strong foundation for becoming a successful surgeon-scientist in any field (Kibbe and LeMaire 2014).

Finally, unless they will have already earned a PhD, students who are strongly contemplating a career in surgical basic science should consider applying to residency programs that provide opportunities to spend dedicated time in a laboratory (see Chap. 15: Choosing a residency program). In such programs, residents usually spend 2 years completing a mentored research fellowship, commonly between their second and third years of clinical training. When visiting and evaluating potential programs, students should seek to learn about the available mentors, the diversity of laboratory options, the accompanying research curriculum, the productivity of residents in terms of publications and presentations, and the program's track record in producing successful surgeon-scientists. Discussions with residents who are currently in the lab or have recently completed their research fellowship can be extremely helpful in determining whether the program is likely to meet the candidate's needs and help them achieve their career goals.

Acknowledgement The author would like to thank Kimberly A. Macellaro, PhD, a member of the Michael E. DeBakey Department of Surgery Research Core at Baylor College of Medicine, for her editorial assistance during the preparation of this manuscript.

References

Bennett LM, Gadlin H, Levine-Finley S. Collaboration and team science: a field guide. Bethesda: National Institutes of Health; 2010.

Economou JS. Gender bias in biomedical research. Surgery. 2014;156(5):1061–5.

Economou JS. Engines of discovery and innovation. Ann Surg. 2016;264(3):405–12.

Folkman J. Francis Daniels Moore: August 17, 1913–November 24, 2001. Biogr Mem Natl Acad Sci. 2006;88:268–82.

Hill GL. Surgeon scientist: adventures in surgical research. Auckland: Random House New Zealand Ltd; 2006.

Kibbe MR, LeMaire SA, editors. Success in academic surgery: basic science. London: Springer; 2014. p. 3–10.

LeMaire SA. Why be an academic surgeon? Impetus and options for the emerging surgeon-scientist. In: Chen H, Kao LS, editors. Success in academic surgery (Part 1). London: Springer; 2012. p. 3–10.

Moore FD. The university in American surgery. Surgery. 1958;44:1–10.

Moore FD. A miracle and a privilege: recounting a half century of surgical advance. Washington, DC: Joseph Henry Press; 1995. p. 382.

National Research Council. Enhancing the effectiveness of team science. Committee on the Science of Team Science. In: Cooke NJ, Hilton ML, editors. Board on behavioral, cognitive, and sensory sciences, division of behavioral and social sciences and education. Washington, DC: The National Academies Press; 2015.

Chapter 4
Global Surgery and Opportunities for Medical Students and Surgical Residents

Anthony Charles, Mamta Swaroop, and Sanjay Krishnaswami

Abstract In the United States and other developed countries, the growing interest in global health among medical students and surgical residents is not just a passing fad, but rather a career choice in academic medicine. Academic Global Surgery (AGS) is becoming a bona fide career track with the goal of improving surgical care delivery in resource-poor settings, through a platform of education, capacity building, and research in addition to clinical care.

4.1 Introduction

In the United States and other developed countries, the growing interest in global health among medical students and surgical residents is not just a passing fad, but rather a career choice in academic medicine (Chin-Quee et al. 2011; Jayaraman et al. 2009). Academic Global Surgery (AGS) is becoming a bona fide career track with the goal of improving surgical care delivery in resource-poor settings, through a platform of education, capacity building, and research in addition to clinical care (Finlayson 2013).

To actively participate and succeed in global surgery, there has to be clarity in motivation and academic aspirations. Some people lend their time to global health for religious reasons or to embark on a journey of self-discovery, while others enjoy the travel and the varied cultural experiences. Although certainly valid reasons for involvement, these alone do not make nor sustain a career in AGS.

A. Charles (✉)
University of North Carolina, Chapel Hill, NC, USA
e-mail: Anthony_charles@med.unc.edu

M. Swaroop
Northwestern Feinberg School of Medicine, Chicago, IL, USA
e-mail: Mamta.swaroop@gmail.com

S. Krishnaswami
Oregon Health Science University, Portland, OR, USA
e-mail: krishnas@ohsu.edu

© Springer International Publishing Switzerland 2017
M.J. Englesbe, M.O. Meyers (eds.), *A How To Guide For Medical Students*,
Success in Academic Surgery, DOI 10.1007/978-3-319-42897-0_4

19

4.2 Getting Started

It is never too early to start to strategically prepare for academic success in global health. Most medical schools now offer month long experiences in global health primarily in Latin America, sub-Saharan Africa, or Southeast Asia. Taking this opportunity is a great way to explore the idea and critically evaluate one's own interests. As importantly, such experiences can involve research projects that lead to presentations and publications at national or international surgical meetings. A number of surgical societies and meetings, such as the Association for Academic Surgery, the Society of University Surgeons, the Academic Surgical Congress and the annual meeting of the American College of Surgeons, now recognize global surgery and have focused sessions in this area just as they do other aspects of surgical science.

For the committed few, spending a year abroad and participating in mentored global health research can be critical to future success. There are organizations that support this endeavor such as the International Clinical Research Fellowship sponsored by the Doris Duke Charitable Foundation and the Fulbright Scholars program. For those with a clear interest in surgery, focusing on such diseases at this stage, though desirable, is not mandatory.

4.3 Postgraduate Training

Choosing a training program that supports their residents' global health interests is very important. In 2011, the General Surgery Residency Review Committee (RRC) of the Accreditation Council for Graduate Medical Education (ACGME) and the American Board of Surgery approved international electives for credit toward residency graduation requirements. After extensive debate on the ways in which international electives could be standardized to ensure consistent educational experience for residents, the surgery RRC approved a set of requirements for such electives (Mitchell et al. 2011; Axt et al. 2013). Given this, there has been an increasing interest within ACGME approved residency programs to offer global surgery opportunities, and a rush to find training sites and partners in developing countries. Successful residencies have the research infrastructure and capacity to build and support an AGS portfolio during residency. Such programs typically demonstrate significant institutional commitment to global health coupled with tangible institutional assets in the developing country of interest. Furthermore, a surgical program that is aligned with a school of public health and offers the opportunity to obtain an M.P.H. may be more desirable.

Many academic surgical residency programs already mandate 1 or 2 years of research time. For those interested in global surgery, the opportunity to undertake clinical outcomes and health services research in a global setting should be seized. Funding for global surgical research is challenging and most surgical programs support these endeavors through fundraising efforts and/or endowments. However, opportunities for external funding do exist. The Fogarty International Center, through the National Institutes of Health, has a Global Health Program for scholars that provides supportive mentorship, research opportunities, and a collaborative research environment for early stage investigators from the U.S. and low- and middle-income countries (LMICs). This funding mechanism can support surgical residents and sets the recipient up for future NIH funding within the global health realm. Because of the rarity of surgeons as applicants for these grants and the new recognition of the role of surgery in public health, the success rate among resident applicants is relatively high. In addition, academic surgical societies such as the Association for Academic Surgery and various specialty-specific societies are beginning to foster the growth of their student and resident members interested in global surgery through competitive research grants (http://www.aasurg.org/awards/fellowship_award_global.php).

More recently, some institutions are now offering AGS fellowships. These have the goals of engaging surgeons in international research, discovery, and training to address the burden of surgical disease, developing the expertise to deliver quality surgical care to developing areas of the world, and promoting the investigative and clinical skills needed in global surgery and humanitarian aid.

4.4 Long-Term: Career Choice, Practice Models, and Departmental Motivations

Upon completion of surgical residency, more than 75 % of all general surgery residents progress to sub-specialization (Charles et al. 2011). Although surgeons across many fields and specialties have engaged in global work, some subspecialties such as trauma/acute care surgery and pediatric surgery may be currently more amenable to an AGS career. This can be because of typical practice configuration, allowing easier sharing of time between overseas partner and home institutions, or because of alignment of the specialty with current priorities in global surgery among other reasons. However, other fields including orthopedic, cardiothoracic, neurosurgery, obstetrics and gynecology, urology, surgical oncology, and plastics/reconstructive surgery are all successfully creating AGS practice models that work in their specific context. It is advisable for the aspiring academic global surgeon to consider feasibility within one's own surgical discipline and remember that health care and research priorities are often determined by the burden of surgical diseases (Charles et al. 2015).

AGS is developing a few different career path models to match the needs of the young surgical faculty and departments. These can be categorized by the allocated time available to be spent in the partnering country and the individual academic global health emphasis (clinical care, education, or research). The most familiar model of time allocation is the use of the surgeon's vacation time, allowing 2–4 weeks per year. This pattern is best suited for participation in focused clinical missions. This model has the advantage that it is not disruptive to a standard surgical practice, but the disadvantage is that it does relatively little to define the surgeon's career trajectory or result in any academic advancement. Another model is the surgeon who is based full-time at the partner institution, with an academic appointment at the home institution. This paradigm allows the surgeon to invest undivided effort in global health work and may perhaps be the most effective model in delivering long-term benefit to the partner institution and region, but it has the disadvantage of rarely being financially supported by the home institution and requiring external funding. More recently, hybrid models have been developed whereby surgeons variably share their time, spending several months in both settings. This has the advantage that the surgeon can act as a living link, bridging the home with the partner institution, allowing sufficient time abroad to coordinate research endeavors, build local research capacity, foster ongoing education and training relationships, and contribute to clinical care while not sacrificing the home surgical networks and practice. Many surgeons are currently engaged in such a mix of activities (Leow et al. 2010).

For many academic surgical chairpersons, the most obvious value of hiring global health faculty is to build global surgical programs that attract the best and brightest trainees, a large proportion of whom are now requesting substantial global health experience and training in their residency programs (Calland et al. 2013). These faculty members are also tasked to guide and mentor interested residents. Aspiring academic global surgeons should recognize the need for departments to stay financially solvent, as global health activity is not a revenue-generating endeavor. This typically forms the basis for initial reluctance by departmental and institutional leadership. Conversely, it is important for chairpersons to acknowledge that global health activity by faculty represents challenging work that supports the academic mission of their department. Increasingly, young faculty recruits with an academic focus in global surgery are being compensated with full salaries comparable to their non-global health counterparts and with protected time to engage in global health work (Tarpley 2013).

4.5 Mentorship

A good mentorship team for any aspiring academic global surgeon is imperative to success. This team can be composed of peers and senior colleagues from any discipline from within or outside your institution. Those *with* experience in low-resource settings can offer guidance in navigating the cultural, clinical and academic nuances unique to such environs while advising on research methodologies appropriate for the particular setting. Mentorship from those *without* specific expertise in global health can still be very valuable in order to offer constructive criticism and objective validation of the methodology and outcomes of your research (Finlayson 2013; Krishnaswami and Swaroop 2016). Both types of mentors can assist with assuring alignment of your work with institutional criteria for academic advancement.

4.6   Conclusion

Global surgery has emerged as an academic surgical discipline and is here to stay. For the student aspiring to a career in AGS, consider short and long-term opportunities that may be available at your home institution and seek out mentors early. Additionally, look for residencies with a proven track record in global surgery. Although some surgical specialties may currently lend themselves more easily to a career in AGS, there are increasing opportunities for global surgery as a faculty career focus across all surgical specialties. To be considered on par with other academic endeavors in surgery, surgeons and trainees must demonstrate rigorous scholarship, successfully study surgical care delivery and health outcomes in low-resource settings, and ideally translate those lessons learned to surgical care delivery at home.

References

Axt J, Nthumba PM, Mwanzia K, et al. Commentary: the role of global surgery electives during residency training: relevance, realities, and regulations. Surgery. 2013;153(3):327–32.

Calland JF, Petroze RT, Abelson J, Kraus E. Engaging academic surgery in global health: challenges and opportunities in the development of an academic track in global surgery. Surgery. 2013;153(3):316–20.

Charles AG, Walker EG, Poley ST, Sheldon GF, Ricketts TC, Meyer AA. Increasing the number of trainees in general surgery residencies: is there capacity? Acad Med. 2011;86(5):599–604.

Charles AG, Samuel JC, Riviello R, Sion MK, Tarpley MJ, Tarpley JL, Olutoye OO, Marcus JR. Integrating global health into surgery residency in the United States. J Surg Educ. 2015;72(4):e88.

Chin-Quee A, White L, Leeds I, MacLeod J, Master VA. Medical student surgery elective in rural Haiti: a novel approach to satisfying clerkship requirements while providing surgical care to an underserved population. World J Surg. 2011;35(4):739–44.

Finlayson SRG. How should academic surgeons respond to enthusiasts of global surgery? Surgery. 2013;153(6):871–2.

http://www.aasurg.org/awards/fellowship_award_global.php

Jayaraman SP, Ayzengart AL, Goetz LH, Ozgediz D, Farmer DL. Global health in general surgery residency: a national survey. J Am Coll Surg. 2009;208(3):426–33.

Krishnaswami S, Swaroop M. Preparing and sustaining your career in academic global surgery. In: Swaroop M, Krishnaswami S, editors. Academic global surgery. Cham: Springer; 2016.

Leow JJ, Kingham TP, Casey KM, Kushner AL. Global surgery: thoughts on an emerging surgical subspecialty for students and residents. J Surg Educ. 2010;67(3):143–8.

Mitchell KB, Tarpley MJ, Tarpley JL, Casey KM. Elective global surgery rotations for residents: a call for cooperation and consortium. World J Surg. 2011;35(12):2617–24.

Tarpley JL. Commentary: an academic track in global surgery. Surgery. 2013;153(3):322–4.

Chapter 5
Personal Wellness and Surgery

Melissa K. Stewart, Michael T. LeCompte, and Kyla P. Terhune

Abstract As an academic surgeon, it's a life of variety—one can aim to master the art of surgery and patient care while also forging the cutting edge of science, dedicating time to mentor others, or working in hospital administration to change care delivery. To succeed in any of these capacities, however, a surgeon must strive for balance, both professionally and personally. Priorities often shift depending on the immediate demands of patients, self, family or others resulting in personal wellbeing often taking a backburner. In the text below, within the context of academic surgery, we will discuss aspects of personal wellness that we have found important through our own experiences or experiences documented by others.

As an academic surgeon, it's a life of variety—one can aim to master the art of surgery and patient care while also forging the cutting edge of science, dedicating time to mentor others, or working in hospital administration to change care delivery. To succeed in any of these capacities, however, a surgeon must strive for balance, both professionally and personally. Priorities often shift depending on the immediate demands of patients, self, family or others resulting in personal wellbeing often taking a backburner. In the text below, within the context of academic surgery, we will discuss aspects of personal wellness that we have found important through our own experiences or experiences documented by others.

First in terms of balance, one must recognize and accept the demands that are inherent to surgery but also celebrate the privilege of being able to care for and impact patients with surgical disease. Surgery is truly a service profession, but it's unique in that there can be some negative consequences. Interventions often carry significant risk, possibly leading to very immediate negative consequences. Not recognizing this and not learning coping skills early in one's residency can lead to anxiety and frustration well into one's career. So, the first step is preparing oneself with very realistic expectations of the demands of the profession. If still up for the

M.K. Stewart (✉) • M.T. LeCompte • K.P. Terhune
Vanderbilt University Medical Center, Nashville, TN, USA
e-mail: Melissa.k.stewart@vanderbilt.edu; Michael.t.lecompte@vanderbilt.edu;
Kyla.terhune@vanderbilt.edu

© Springer International Publishing Switzerland 2017
M.J. Englesbe, M.O. Meyers (eds.), *A How To Guide For Medical Students,*
Success in Academic Surgery, DOI 10.1007/978-3-319-42897-0_5

challenge, read on. The following discussion is intended to aid you in achieving balance as you shape and navigate your career.

5.1 Set Your Own Personal Priorities

To navigate the personal and professional complexities of surgery in an effort to attain wellness, one must set personal priorities—and these can only be set by you, as they are unique to you—best set in medical school and in residency. It requires introspection: understanding who and what you are; this includes appreciating your talents, pursuing your passions and accepting your strengths and weaknesses. Is family a major priority? What kinds of problems do you like to solve? What's your best working environment? What do you want to accomplish? Is your mission to be a busy surgeon practicing and providing care in a small rural community? A global surgeon in sub-Saharan Africa performing outcomes research? A surgeon who gets to golf every Wednesday? An academic surgeon with a basic science laboratory in a major city? A part-time surgeon with a beach bungalow? Be brutally honest with yourself so you can frame your decision-making around it. This allows you to develop a mission that encompasses your goals, giving meaning and a framework for training.

5.2 Maintain Yourself Mentally and Physically, Through Exercise and Regular Medical Care

The initial prevention strategy and solution to attaining balance involves "me" time—not just "me in the bathtub with a good book" time, but regular time working on your own physical, emotional and mental well-being. All too often, when life gets busy and stressed, one's own personal time is the first to be eliminated. To avoid this trend, try to remember the following tips.

- **Be grateful, you're pretty lucky to be where you are.** A survey noted that by simply maintaining a positive outlook and embracing a philosophy that stresses work-life balance, rates of burnout were decreased (Shanafelt et al. 2012). Experience also suggests that the simple act of being grateful, expressing this to others or keeping your own record of things for which you are grateful, significantly increases job satisfaction.
- **Exercise regularly, even if just a little bit.** Beyond emotional wellbeing, it is also important to prioritize and optimize physical health. Surgeons who engage in aerobic and muscle strengthening activities had improved quality of life scores (Irani et al. 2005). Some surgeons note that exercise programs that emphasize bursts of exercise regularly, such as interval running, interval exercise programs

or even vigorously walking stairs for 20–30 min a day, are easier to maintain and are more conducive to the work schedule of a surgeon or trainee.

- **Get your own physician.** Establishing a relationship with a primary care physician and attaining appropriate preventive medical care is of utmost importance. Surveys indicate that only 46.2% of surgeons are regularly evaluated by their primary care physician. Surgeons who received care in the last 12 months were more likely to be compliant with health screening recommendations and boasted superior overall and physical quality of life scores (Shanafelt et al. 2012).
- **Recognize that you are human.** Just as important to seeking medical care for physical ailments, promptly attending to mental health concerns is paramount. Depression and substance abuse are realistic concerns, even for those who might consider themselves immune. Sadly, secondary to lack of recognition or to concern for repercussions, surgeons are often reluctant to seek psychological or psychiatric assistance. As an example, only 26% of surgeons with suicidal ideation sought professional help. The same study noted that the reluctance to seek help was based on the concern that it may adversely affect their professional life (Shanafelt et al. 2011). Another reason for reluctance may be perceived lack of time to dedicate to psychiatric care. Though time may be scarce, it is evident that seeking care will allow for improved personal wellbeing, more robust and fruitful personal relationships and likely more effective and efficient professional endeavors.

5.3   Nurture Your Relationships with Others

Relationships not only provide a crucial support system but also function to provide a meaningful context to life. A gross majority of screened surgeons reported that spousal relationships were adversely affected by the demands of work (Colletti et al. 2000). How do we fix this? Is the solution to decrease the demands of the job? This may be part of the remedy. The majority of surgery residents, 71%, noted an improvement in the quality of relationships following restriction of work hours (Irani et al. 2005). Generally, however, we do not have full control over professional demands and work hour restrictions don't extend into practice. The more plausible answer is prioritization of specific time to devote to relationship development. This also holds true for familial relationships.

- **Spend quality time, when quantity may not be possible.** Regardless of the relationship, be it with parents, significant others, friends or children, it is imperative that the time spent together is prioritized, with minimal external distractions, even if for a shorter period of time. You must be totally devoted, both physically and mentally, to make the most of the encounter. Multitasking or being absent minded will be poorly received and will compromise the time that was set aside for relationship building.

- **Remind others that you're thankful they're with you.** The relationship most often taken for granted is that of a significant other, such as a spouse or partner. Arming these individuals with awareness prospectively is helpful. If you are entering surgery residency or accepting an academic surgery position with a significant other or family by your side, significant others need to be fully educated on the process and be aware of the stresses and strains. Your relationships will have a higher likelihood of prospering if all involved parties 'get-it'. Then, never forget to express gratitude frequently–for the support given during one's training and profession, so that family members recognize that they too help support patient care indirectly by directly supporting you.
- **Make it to as many of the "big" events as you can…and the small ones too.** Prioritize and attend family events as often as able. Coordinating family vacations, making it to weddings, family reunions, etc., are important. One of the authors tried to schedule vacations around children's birthdays during residency to ensure that she had dedicated, unchallenged time on these particular days. However, attending big events may not always be possible, and you should be prepared to have an honest conversation about why you can't make it sometimes. Moreover, attempt to make the small events seem big—attempt to elevate helping with chores or homework by being mentally present. Also, work as a team with your fellow residents and future partners—if you support them, they are more likely to support you.
- **Create an umbrella of mentors.** It can be dangerous to seek a single mentor and focus on this relationship exclusively. It may lead to disappointment, inappropriate situations or exclusion of other potentially meaningful interactions. Instead, seek multiple mentors for different aspects of your professional and personal life—economists have known for a long time that diversification increases the value of your portfolio. The same holds true for mentors.

5.4   Choose a Residency Program/Faculty Appointment That Will Allow You to Honor Your Priorities

Similar to the discussion above regarding personal and family considerations, specific actions and prioritization must occur at the professional level to successfully attain work-life balance. The initial professional consideration occurs prior to accepting a residency or faculty position.

- **Define your own personal vision or mission, or at least your priorities.** Your priorities will change as you age, but it's important to establish your own vision of what you want to "be" or accomplish. As noted above, even if you are undecided about *which* surgical specialty or fellowship you want to pursue, think about *where* you want to live, *where* you want to work, *who* you want to be with and how you see your life years down the road. Consider your strengths and weaknesses and enlist mentors to aid in the discussion. It is vital to seek out an environment with mentors who want to invest in your growth as a physician and help you develop your career and support you personally. A good mentor will push you to advance and be productive but will also be there to get you out of a rut or a difficult time. Don't have a vision? Then list your most important priorities *in your life now* and be honest with yourself about these (You don't have to necessarily be honest with others).

- **Interview and rank residency programs with your priorities in mind.** Your outlined vision, mission or priorities should assist you as you make decisions regarding interviewing and ranking programs. When you interview, consider a residency that aligns with who and what you want to "be". After all, you will spend a significant amount of time in residency, and it is worthwhile to remember that your life does not start at the end of residency but continues while within it. You won't enjoy every minute you spend in residency (or any job for that matter). However, residency is a unique experience that can be fun, rewarding, exciting and memorable, and you should seek out an environment that fosters more fulfillment than dissatisfaction.
- **Choose your residency and fellowship... and everything else with your priorities in mind.** Having your priorities established, use these as a roadmap or guide in every decision that you make for the rest of your life. As you advance, pay attention to what realms of surgery—administration, education, science and/ or operative and clinical management—you find most meaningful and gratifying. Additionally, you must carefully choose and limit your extracurricular academic activities based on these priorities. Avoid trying to be an active, contributing member of all pertinent academic societies or all clubs or all anything. Pick a few things that align with your priorities and focus on these.

5.5   Seek a Higher Purpose or Belief System—Even if Is Just Trying to Improve the Human Condition

Disclaimer: this is not an endorsement of any religion—it's an endorsement of thinking beyond yourself, which many would argue is the purpose of medicine. Spirituality can be defined as the sense of meaning, truth and purpose in regards to the concept of the divine and the integration of these principles into life (Seybold and Hill 2001). Seeking a higher purpose can be improvement of humanity or simply a sense of "goodness" or altruism. Integration of spiritual health practices, in addition to standard medical treatment, has been demonstrated in multiple studies to improve overall health and satisfaction among patients (Daaleman 2004; Best et al. 2013; Pargament et al. 2004) as well as benefit physician wellbeing (Seybold and Hill 2001; Yi et al. 2006; Doolittle et al. 2013).

- **Practice mindfulness.** Many are drawn to the medical field as a profession that exemplifies caring for others and the betterment of humanity. However, these feelings can also be drowned out by stress, fatigue, loneliness and undesired medical outcomes. A gradual decline of empathy, compassion and altruism has been well documented during residency and is correlated with burnout (Gleichgerrcht and Decety 2013). In a high-paced job such as surgery, slowing down and practicing short bursts of meditation, deep-breathing or even concentration can help one to gather thoughts and avoid anxiety or pressure that might lead to being overwhelmed. Practicing "mindfulness," or being conscious of both internal and external experiences, helps one with general awareness. It is easy to find oneself angry or frustrated by the 2 am patient consult or page for Tylenol; however, it is important to take a moment to comprehend that you have the responsibility to relieve the suffering of someone in need, and this is a noble task.

- **Connect with others. And be honest.** Finding time to connect with your coworkers on a deeper level can be difficult; however, remember that they are going through the same struggles. Residency training environments that foster regular discussion of professional successes, failures and difficult experiences in a protected environment have been shown to promote professional development and a sense of collegial community (Rabow and McPhee 2001). This discussion allows trainees to see that they are not alone in struggling with the pressures of a stressful environment and their own limitations in the modern medical climate. Routine practice of this form of discussion, in turn, was shown to promote a renewed sense of duty and empathy towards patients (Rabow and McPhee 2001).
- **Spend time reflecting.** Taking time for personal and professional reflection has also been shown to be beneficial. Reflective writing, journaling or blogging has been demonstrated to improve empathy, humanism and professionalism among residents as well as reduce levels of stress (Rabow and McPhee 2001; Bernard et al. 2012). Specifically, being able to express frustration, anger or personal shortcomings in writing helps one cope with these emotions and helps provides a stability and frame of reference for dealing with similar situations in the future (Rabow and McPhee 2001). It is also important to capture moments of triumph, satisfaction and meaningful patient interactions. Save thank-you cards and emails. This allows one to return to these moments in the future and use them in times where they feel their confidence, empathy, compassion or sense of humanity dwindling.
- **Seek out others with similar beliefs (but don't forget to learn from those with different beliefs).** Spirituality, in the context of religious practice, can offer access to supportive networks and relationships during times of illness and stress. One study demonstrated rates of significant depressive symptoms in 25 % of residents administered the validated 10- Item Center for Epidemiologic Studies Depression Scale (Yi et al. 2006). Residents who reported poor spiritual wellbeing or who had a "non-designated religious affiliation" were at higher risk for depressive symptoms. As many residents must re-locate and move away from communities and congregations to pursue residency or fellowship training, this may leave them vulnerable to spiritual health decline during their training. Thus, for these individuals, it is important to re-establish connection in a spiritual community early during their training.

5.6 If You Want to Have a Family, Have a Family! but Prepare Yourself with Knowledge

This statement is directed to men and women alike. Starting a family in residency is not uncommon. Research completed in 2013 showed that 41 % of males and 35 % of females will have a child during residency (Smith et al. 2013). Although this should be able to be accommodated in any professional working environment in this century, there still may be stigmas that exist. If these bother you, it may be helpful to search for programs that have demonstrated successful navigation of this process, of which there are many. Regardless, it is important to arm yourself with knowledge. Although some pregnancies are surprises (and some pregnancies are unexpectedly complicated), planning to the degree that is possible will help ensure enough time off, salary and benefits during the time off, with maximum time away but minimum disruption of training which can lead to a healthier baby and healthier and happier parents. Additionally, it allows for one to maximize one's financial and support systems, two things that are required for ongoing sustenance during training, especially with children.

- **Know the laws in your state.** The Family Medical Leave Act (FMLA) is *not* the same thing as maternity or paternity leave (United States Department of Labor, http www dol govwhdfmlaindex htm). Companies (e.g. hospital employers, as in residency) are not required to provide maternity or paternity leave, leave usually thought of as paid leave with benefits. FMLA is different—it is up to 12 weeks of time that runs concurrent with any paid or unpaid leave, and it essentially just means that you won't be fired during a specified period if the circumstance is defined under FMLA. Some states have eligibility for additional time. However, many employees in the first year of their employment at a new company are not eligible for FMLA. What does this mean? This means that, theoretically, under a certain set of circumstances (e.g. in the first year of training), one might be in a situation with no FMLA, no maternity/paternity leave, and very few sick days accumulated, potentially leaving him or her in an absence which is unpaid and without benefits. Although not all pregnancies are planned, a degree of knowledge and planning is important when possible to minimize this additional surprise.
- **Know the training requirements of your certifying board.** At the end of one's training, he or she wants to be board-eligible. For example, at the time of writing this, the American Board of Surgery (ABS) has much more flexibility than it has in the past, but it is still limited compared to what one might receive as a primary employee in another organization. One needs to have 48 weeks of clinical (non-vacation) training per year, averaged in the first 3 years and the final 2 years in order to be eligible at the end of training to sit for the qualifying exam (QE). If one has a medical condition himself or herself (pregnancy included for her), one may request an additional 2 weeks of non-clinical time in a particular year. Additionally, because of averaging, any resident can "bank" vacation time within

the first 3 years and the final 2 years of training to the extent permitted by the program. Moreover, one may apply for approval to extend training to a sixth clinical year when needed to make up missed time. Please note, ABS policies change periodically, so please check the current status. The main point is that being eligible from a training standpoint needs to be considered separately from time away allowed by an employer.

- **Know the benefit structure.** As noted above, it is important to know from your primary institution (where your contract is) what the regulations are regarding whether one would receive salary and/or benefits during a prolonged absence. These are typically available on institutional websites and contracts are required to be available at the time of the interview.

With all of the scary legal language out of the way, having a family is possible and can be incredibly fulfilling with the right knowledge, support structure (someone with flexibility for patient care and childcare) and desire.

5.7   Conclusion

Through this chapter, we hoped to convey the importance of focusing on wellbeing during your journey into residency and future career as an academic surgeon. We hope to equip and encourage you as you seek out a rich and fulfilling profession and to avoid the common perils and pitfalls that can lead one astray. Not every strategy will work for everyone, and the list is not exhaustive. Each of the authors has been encouraged to "get in the habit of making good habits"—this is valid for both in the workplace and at home. Start by choosing one or two areas to focus on and make them priority with regular practice.

We will leave you with this—Teddy Roosevelt once said "Far and away the best prize that life has to offer is the chance to work hard at work worth doing". It's a tough road, but with balance, it can be a sustained road—and we can think of no work more worth doing.

References

Bernard AW, Gorgas D, Greenberger S, Jacques A, Khandelwal S. The use of reflection in emergency medicine education. Acad Emerg Med. 2012;19:978–82.

Best M, Butow P, Olver I. Spiritual support of cancer patients and the role of the doctor. Support Care Cancer. 2013;22:1333–9.

Colletti LM, Mulholland MW, Sonnad SS. Perceived obstacles to career success for women in academic surgery. Arch Surg. 2000;135:972–7.

Daaleman TP. Religion, spirituality, and health status in geriatric outpatients. Ann Fam Med. 2004;2:49–53.

Doolittle BR, Windish DM, Seelig CB. Burnout, coping, and spirituality among internal medicine resident physicians. J Grad Med Educ. 2013;5:257–61.

Gleichgerrcht E, Decety J. Empathy in clinical practice: How individual dispositions, gender, and experience moderate empathic concern, burnout, and emotional distress in physicians. PLoS ONE. 2013;8, e61526.

Irani JL et al. Surgical residents' perceptions of the effects of the ACGME duty hour requirements 1 year after implementation. Surgery. 2005;138:246–53.

Pargament KI, Koenig HG, Tarakeshwar N, Hahn J. Religious coping methods as predictors of psychological, physical and spiritual outcomes among medically Ill elderly patients: a Two-year longitudinal study. J Health Psychol. 2004;9:713–30.

Rabow MW, McPhee SJ. Doctoring to heal: fostering well-being among physicians through personal reflection. West J Med. 2001;174:66–9.

Seybold KS, Hill PC. The role of religion and spirituality in mental and physical health. Curr Dir Psychol Sci. 2001;10:21–4.

Shanafelt TD et al. Special report: suicidal ideation among American surgeons. Arch Surg. 2011;146:54–62.

Shanafelt TD et al. Avoiding burnout. Ann Surg. 2012;255:625–33.

Smith C, Galante JM, Pierce JL, Scherer LA. The surgical residency baby boom: changing patterns of childbearing during residency over a 30-year span. J Grad Med Educ. 2013;5:625–9.

The American Board of Surgery. Booklet of Information: Surgery. http://www.absurgery.org/xfer/BookletofInfo-Surgery.pdf

United States Department of Labor. Wage and Hour Division: Family and Medical Leave Act. http:www.dol.govwhdfmlaindex.htm

Yi MS et al. Religion, spirituality, and depressive symptoms in primary care house officers. Ambul Pediatr. 2006;6:84–90.

Chapter 6
Perspective of a Program Director

Jahnavi Srinivasan and Keith Delman

Abstract Once a student has made the choice to embark on a career in surgery, the next step is to figure out how to choose the training program that is the right fit. Just as each applicant is unique, so is each program. That being said, all surgical residencies value a certain set of core characteristics in common. This chapter gives the perspective of a surgical program director on qualities that make for a successful surgery resident.

Once a student has made the choice to embark on a career in surgery, the next step is to figure out how to choose the training program that is the right fit. Just as each applicant is unique, so is each program. That being said, all surgical residencies value a certain set of core characteristics in common. This chapter gives the perspective of a surgical program director on qualities that make for a successful surgery resident.

6.1 Start from a Place of Certainty

Students should first ask themselves why they are choosing a career in surgery. If the student does not have a visceral answer that he or she would be comfortable writing into a personal statement or declaring at an interview, it is perhaps wise to rethink this professional choice. This is the first opportunity in the career of a student that impacts future success, and the applicant should be mindful that a happy and productive career first stems from making the choice to do what one actually enjoys.

If taking care of surgical pathology in and out of the operating room doesn't inherently appeal to the student, a life in surgery may not be the correct choice. Prospective trainees often mention, with a hint of irritation, that they dislike getting

J. Srinivasan (✉) • K. Delman
Emory University School of Medicine, Atlanta, GA, USA
e-mail: jsrini2@emory.edu; kdelman@emory.edu

© Springer International Publishing Switzerland 2017
M.J. Englesbe, M.O. Meyers (eds.), *A How To Guide For Medical Students*,
Success in Academic Surgery, DOI 10.1007/978-3-319-42897-0_6

35

advice not to choose surgery if there is anything else they could possibly enjoy. While it is certainly true that the aspirational and dedicated nature of the medical profession results in significant sacrifice no matter what the specialty, procedural specialties like surgery have a distinctly unique impact on lifestyle and work hours simply by nature of the job.

When processing cautionary advice from attending surgeons, it's useful to remember that program directors were all once applying and interviewing for surgical residencies too. They all remember the visceral emotion and rational calculation that went into their own decisions. To the students, it may seem like these poised, grey-haired faculty giving them career advice are anachronisms- a remnant of pre-80 h-work week ideals that don't apply to the modern surgical era. However, once the surgeon has made an incision, he or she owns the postoperative consequences to the patient that may run the gamut from an unplanned reoperation to a discussion about medical futility and palliation. It is the psychological and physical burden of the surgical profession that leads its actual practitioners to caution the eager apprentice. If a student has not truly thought through these common scenarios, and worked through the impact on his or her psyche, reconsideration of why they've made the career choice may be required. As discouraging as this may seem, the student should remember that the goal of any program is to accept candidates with the greatest chance of success in their training. An articulation of these considerations, and the subsequent decision to still choose a career in surgery illustrates maturity and an undeterred desire that reassures programs about their choice of the applicant.

6.2 Demonstrate Your Ability to Succeed at Fundamentals

Once the student has affirmed his or her surgical career choice, the next step in the process is figuring out how to find THE program at which to train. It's easiest to start with discussing the traits that all programs desire in a trainee. Every surgical program, at its most basic, looks to produce graduates who are technically adept surgeons at any hour, under any amount of pressure, however inconvenient the situation. This sounds straight forward enough, but students should remember that programs all have their own histories of trainees who have succeeded and those who have failed. Applicants will therefore be scrutinized with the goal of recreating the success stories and avoiding the failures. Qualities that demonstrate an ability to successfully overcome setbacks will be seen as a surrogate for surgical success and should be highlighted for any program to which a student applies.

One of the characteristics important to all programs is a demonstration of academic success. When looking at surveys of independent and academic surgical residency programs, it has held true that USMLE scores significantly correlate to a program's willingness to offer an applicant an interview and match that applicant to their program (Dort et al. 2015; Stain et al. 2013). While criticisms of standardized testing as a proxy for knowledge are recognized, it is certainly true that success with these exams is still viewed as a marker for students who will have less difficulty mastering a broad fund of knowledge. During training, surgical residents will continue to take the American Board of Surgery In-training exam (ABSITE), and a demonstration of prior success on standardized tests does reassure programs that this is a realm in which a prospective trainee will be less likely to struggle. In fact, USMLE scores are used at many programs as one of the filters for evaluating applications that will be considered for interviews. For students who did not perform at the mean on USMLE Step 1, showing a substantial improvement on USMLE Step 2 demonstrates several things to programs; particularly that there is not a pattern of performing poorly on standardized testing and that the applicant has the ability to rally when faced with a setback.

An excellent surrogate for outstanding results on standardized examinations and grades in preclinical classwork is success in other endeavors, such as sports, service organizations, music and the arts or other significant accomplishments. These successes generally require hard work, organization, frequently reflect intrinsic leadership skills and often predict success in other areas of one's life. Undoubtedly, national recognition for a hobby, sport or musical pursuit is something that will catch the eye of a program director and potentially mitigate grades that are slightly less than outstanding.

Clinical transcripts do matter, and programs will particularly scrutinize a student's performance on their surgery rotation and surgical sub-internship rotation. Additionally, success in all clerkships is generally scrutinized as a surrogate for interpersonal effectiveness and the ability to translate knowledge into clinical acumen. Despite a consideration of all clinical experiences, surgical residencies generally expect that individuals truly interested in surgery will naturally show themselves at their best when on a rotation that represents an experience akin to their future profession. The ability to distinguish oneself on a surgical rotation goes beyond studied knowledge and demonstrates 'in the trenches' ability to put that knowledge to use in a functional way. Some important qualities that have an intangible, gestalt quality are best evaluated by a student's clinical performance because the human element, which is critical to this profession, bears more heavily into play. An applicant's personality, professionalism, bedside manner, team integration, work ethic, and intraoperative demeanor are all evaluated on a surgery rotation in a way that no formal test can quantify.

6.3   Prove Your Rigor

Surgery is a profession that, by its nature, requires a physical and mental toughness. After programs have set their thresholds for the basics of an application (USMLE scores and rotation grades) they will look for other signs in the application that demonstrate an applicant's perseverance and rigor. The specific 'what' involved in doing that can vary, but a common example accepted amongst surgeons who have tried to catalogue markers in individuals who have excelled in residency is being an athlete of distinction. Athletes will often set a demanding training regimen at the sacrifice of personal time in order focus on attaining their set goal. They will over-come personal deficiencies by practicing at the task until they have hit a level of perfection. The analogy extends further in cases of team sports, where the entire effort is crippled if members cannot work with one another toward a common effort. As noted in the prior section, the same can be said of individuals who have built on an effort from scratch to high levels of achievement, be it the principle investigator in an elite science lab, the humanitarian who is the force behind a non-governmental organization (NGO), or the business-minded individual who starts a successful company. Life and work experiences that mimic qualities that lead to success in surgery will be taken seriously as an indication that a prospective trainee will have the initiative to be self-driven and not spoon fed through training.

6.4   Have an Honest Sense of Your Career Goals

While it is true that certain qualities are valued in common by all programs, the degree to which different characteristics are encouraged and coveted varies. Some programs focus on high volume broad general surgical training with the goal of producing the work force of surgeons who will shoulder the burden of clinical care and service to the greater population. Some programs seek surgeons intended for academics, building mandatory research time into their program, and having the expectation that fellowship specialization will follow core training. Many programs are a mix along the aforementioned spectrum of clinical versus academic. Certainly the exposure an individual receives during training can completely alter the course of one's planned future, but by in large, most people know which category of train-ing into which they will fall when they complete medical school. By embracing the arena in which one excels and choosing a program whose training goals are compat-ible with one's future goals, both the applicant and program will be happier. Surrounding oneself with mentors and colleagues who are of a similar training mindset provides a better fit and leaves less room for internal and external conflict during surgical residency. More than that, opportunities to pursue one's career inter-ests are more likely found at places that are inherently geared toward fostering and developing those goals already.

To this end, one's stated career goals should match their resume. Claiming to desire a future in laboratory research in the absence of any bench research and pub-lications will call into question the sincerity of such statements. Programs want to see that there is evidence and substance behind professed ambitions. This is an area where strong letters of recommendation from surgeons who have extensively worked with a student over lukewarm letters from surgeons with only a superficial knowledge of a prospective trainee can make a big difference for the applicant.

6.5   Be Your Best Advocate

Surgery is not a passive sport, and applicants who are not active participants in their destiny may not end up satisfied with the end result. Once students have decided upon a surgical career, identification of a surgical mentor for career advice and planning is critical. If that mentor does not actively support their mentee, looking for a more proactive and engaged advisor is not just suggested, it is mandatory. Faculty, particularly program directors and chairs, are exceedingly busy, and it is the student's responsibility to reengage their surgical attendings as needed for support in the process. Failure to distinguish oneself in a sea of other applicants lies more squarely on the shoulders of the student than the faculty, whom often have several students queued up for whom they have to write letters of recommendation and provide advice.

Just as important as it is to highlight one's strengths, knowledge of one's weaknesses can preempt an undesirable match result. Students should be proactive about soliciting feedback, even when negative, from faculty mentors so they are best prepared for how the are honestly seen by those likely to evaluate them. The ability to process criticism constructively is critical for all surgeons, and starting this process early on can only help the applicant develop a healthy sense of introspection that can be used in the future to negotiate the hurdles that surgical training invariably brings. Open acknowledgement of one's weaknesses is requisite in anyone who wants to make progress, and it is the contradictory qualities of supreme confidence mixed with ready humility that often distinguish practitioners of surgery from other professions.

6.6   It Is Truly a Match

One of the best ways for an applicant and program to know if they are meant for one another is through extended exposure. Once an applicant has settled upon their path of training, they should look at the list of programs throughout the country and decide which of those programs meet their requirements. Applicants will tend to have insight into their home institution because of the amount of time they have spent on rotations there as students. They get to know staff and residents better than their counterparts from other institutions, and thus way the pros and cons with a greater quantity of information than an 'outsider' might. If an institution inside or outside of one's geographic region appears to meet many of an applicant's training requirements, it is not unreasonable to do an away rotation at that institution to develop 'insider' knowledge of how the program functions. It is important to note that "away rotations" are not required and certainly should not be perceived as "auditions". On the contrary, they are an opportunity for a student to gather important exposure to the mundane aspects of a residency program. Talking with the trainees at a program, and watching how they interact with one another can inform an applicant by volumes about their likelihood of fitting into a program as well. Thus, it is important to take advantage of social nights arranged during interview time to get to know the residents. On the program side, the existing residents are certainly evaluating the students during these sessions to get a sense about 'fit' with their team. Applicants should heavily weigh what their instinct tells them about fit in a particular environment.

Outside of USMLE scores, geographic location of medical school has been shown to be another predictor of match, with most residents matching into training within their medical school's region. Certainly, part of the reason for that is that programs within a similar geographic region tend to have a greater familiarity with one another's residencies. One must also consider that programmatic culture is influence at least in part by geographic region as well, and thus trainee personality 'fits' may be better when people stay within the region from which they went to school.

Ultimately, intellectual honesty with oneself is critical to be happy in this profession. Students should remember that they are who they are, and trying to fit a square peg into a round hole is never going to result in success. Budding surgeons excel when they enjoy what they are doing. Students who make their match process deliberate rather than defaulting into the path of least resistance are the most likely to end up in a happy and secure place.

6.7 You Are Who You Are

Finally, the student should not lose sight of who they are. One of the most critical aspects of matching is recognizing your own learning style and identifying the environment in which you will thrive. The aforementioned traits and criteria by which you will be benchmarked are critical two-way assessment tools that will help a student and a residency program identify appropriate "matches" who will thrive in any given program. Given this, it is vital that the student be honest about who they are, their strengths and weaknesses, and their learning style. It is not uncommon, when being asked for advice about applying for a residency, that a student will ask, "what can I do to make myself a stronger applicant." There is very little that one can actively do in a short period of time (1 year or less) to truly change their application, but instead, the applicant should focus on the points that were highlighted previously—be their best advocate, highlight and understand their strengths and goals, and be willing to acknowledge their weaknesses and how they mitigate them. Finally, it is imperative that the student understands where their passion lies. Passion cannot be faked and if the applicant is truly passionate about surgery and the care of patients, it will be evident from their interview. Interviewers will find it infectious to speak with the student and will share in their passion, at least momentarily while engaged. It may not mean that the applicant's passion meshes with a particular program, but as long as the student is honest about it, he or she will end up with the perfect match.

References

Dort JM, Trickey AW, Kallies KJ, Joshi AR, Sidwell RA, Jarman BT. Applicant characteristics associated with selection for ranking at independent surgery residency programs. J Surg Educ. 2015;72(6), e123.

Stain SC, Hiatt JR, Ata A, Ashley SW, Roggin KK, Potts JR, Moore RA, Galante JM, Britt LD, Deveney KE, Ellison EC. Characteristics of highly ranked applicants to general surgery residency programs. JAMA Surg. 2013;148(5):413–7.

Part II
Building a Portfolio for Success

Chapter 7
Working on Yourself: Intangibles of a Successful Surgery Resident

Amir A. Ghaferi

Abstract Self-actualization is the key to success as a surgical resident. Students who have chosen a future in surgery are a motivated, eager, and confident group. The importance of continual self improvement is paramount to success. As such, leadership, communication, and resilience are three traits that provide room for such growth. This chapter will provide insights and advice on how to "work on yourself."

7.1 The Goal: Develop a Strong Foundation in Leadership, Communication, and Resilience

Students choosing to pursue a career in surgery have self-selected as future leaders. Surgery is a contact sport with surgeons, nurses, scrub technicians, and patients occupying the same arena. They are all fighting the same opponent—surgical disease. This is a team of professionals that are often thrown together during a critically important episode of care. The situation demands that they are cohesive, confident, and focused. No one ever conquers a surgical disease without a surgeon who is an effective leader, a master communicator, and resilient in the face of adversity.

Leadership, communication, and resilience are the three traits that are the marker of a successful surgical resident and future surgical leader.

A.A. Ghaferi (✉)
Department of Surgery, University of Michigan, Ann Arbor, MI, USA
e-mail: aghaferi@med.umich.edu

© Springer International Publishing Switzerland 2017
M.J. Englesbe, M.O. Meyers (eds.), *A How To Guide For Medical Students,*
Success in Academic Surgery, DOI 10.1007/978-3-319-42897-0_7

7.1.1 Leadership Development

What are the core values every leader possesses? The following are neither all encompassing nor developed by consensus—respect, integrity, authenticity, service, humility, and wisdom. It is incumbent upon you to seek experiences during medical school to foster these traits or develop them de novo. Leadership is not an inherent characteristic. It requires deliberate awareness of oneself and always seeking to improve.

Surgical residents are recognized leaders in the hospital. Surgical residents find themselves as the "go-to" physician in the hospital whenever there is a crisis. The respect garnered by surgical chief residents is an important responsibility that they carry with them daily. However, there are also anecdotes of surgical chief residents being ineffective due to their leadership style. Leadership, practiced at its best, is the art and science of calling to the hearts and minds of others. It is engaging others in an enterprise of sound strategic focus, where they experience a sense of ownership, of making a difference, of being valued and adding value. These attributes are essential to the cohesiveness needed in the healthcare setting to care for the sickest and most complex patients.

As a result, surgery program directors are aware of the need for selecting medical students who have demonstrated the ability to lead others by example, by inspiring, and by learning. While some leaders are born, the majority must seek development opportunities or are a product of the circumstances they find themselves in. The question remains how to acquire the necessary experiences and skills to become an effective leader.

First, one should identify a mentor or individual who's leadership style resonates with him or her. Ideally, this individual holds defined leadership roles, such as an administrative chief resident, leader of a clinical program, division chief, or director of a research program. Observing the animal in his or her habitat be educational and inspirational. Pay attention to the short term goals set by the leader and how the team is motivated to achieve excellence and success. Beyond the short term, observe how the leader outlines a vision for the group. A vision gives everyone engaged something to strive for and a larger context within which to plan and set strategy. It provides everyone with an essential sense of direction and purpose, whether it is which part of the task to own, or more profoundly, who and what the team is striving to become.

Second, discover an organization that resonates with your personal values and beliefs, such as a fraternity or sorority, charity group, religious organization, or educational mission. Engage in the group by organizing an event, keynote lecture, symposium, group meeting, workshop, or outreach activity. The key is to be invested in the success and growth of the group. Substance over quantity is key here. Being a member in multiple organizations as a follower demonstrates the ability to attend meetings and eat a free lunch. Being a leader requires courage and dedication. The seven acts of courage laid out by Robert Staub in *The Heart of Leadership* include:

1. The courage to dream and put forth that dream.
2. The courage to see current reality.

3. The courage to confront.
4. The courage to be confronted.
5. The courage to learn and grow.
6. The courage to be vulnerable
7. The courage to act.

Finally, be flexible in your leadership style and seek continuous feedback on how to improve. This requires seeking feedback from peers, superiors, and juniors. Remember, seeking a pat on the back is not the goal here. It is important to create an environment where honest feedback is given without fear of offending you, creating an awkward work environment, or worry about reprimand. A proven method of doing this is using anonymous feedback tools such as "360 evaluations" or online survey tools such as Qualtrics. This is becoming a widespread and accepted practice in medicine, especially surgery. There are many valuable resources such as books and online tools that also provide instruments for assessing your leadership style, your individual blind spots in leadership, and methods for improving daily.

7.1.2 Communication Skills

The ability to communicate with peers, consultants, and patients is of utmost importance to a career in surgery. We are often faced with difficult, complex patients with multidisciplinary pathology. Surgeons are expected to be the clinical champion for many patients by synthesizing input from multiple providers, the patients themselves, and family members. The ability to communicate important facts and views is an invaluable attribute of a successful surgeon. It is naïve to see this as an intrinsic trait of any individual. It requires refining throughout the course of one's training.

This begins during residency where an intern is viewed as a reporter of information. This is encapsulated in the notes that they write as communication to other providers and verbal communication to patients, families, and superiors. Toward the end of internship, surgical house officers are expected to begin synthesizing information into relevant pieces that explain the clinical story of the patient in a clear and concise manner. The learning curve is steep and there is always room for improvement. During the ensuing years, residents are expected create a more cohesive interpretation of objective and subjective data elicited from the patient, providers, physical examinations, and laboratory and radiologic studies.

Building and honing these skills is not a simple task. Much like leadership, it is a lifelong endeavor that requires hard work and a willingness to adapt, grow, and accept feedback. The following are some strategies on how to begin working on communication skills during medical school.

First, writing is one of the most important skills that all professionals should maintain and cultivate during their careers. The most obvious times that surgeons need to be effective writers are through operative notes, clinic notes, and letters to consulting physicians. In academic surgery, one of the most recognizable currencies is peer reviewed manuscripts. Each of these forms of writing require the ability to communicate plainly and succinctly without missing important details.

Medical students have the opportunity to write clinic and progress notes. This may be viewed as grunt work, and it is if there is no feedback loop. Students must seek meaningful feedback from other students, junior and senior residents, and faculty. The most powerful feedback comes during these formative years of training. Entering residency with sharpened writing skills will prove to be a valuable asset.

Manuscripts provide additional opportunity to practice a different type of writing. While the research opportunities vary across medical schools, there are many chances to write case reports, viewpoints, and review articles. Mentors must be carefully sought out to find valuable experiences. Manuscript preparation is very much like patient care. It requires identifying a problem or question, gathering data, analyzing and interpreting facts, drawing conclusions from that information, and finally communicating it through writing. These skills require thoughtful practice and proper mentorship.

Another important method of sharing research brings to light the second form of communication that is vital to a successful surgical resident/surgeon—speaking. Increasingly, local and national meetings are encouraging the participation of medical students in their programs. These meetings provide an exceptional occasion for students to gain exposure to high level research discussions, present their work and gain insight from others about their research, and to meet new people from medical schools and surgical residencies around the country. The ability to access these types of events depends on the environment of the medical school and its different departments. Seeking the input or mentorship of people outside your home institution is also encouraged.

7.1.3 Resilience

Resilience is a hot topic and buzz word in both business and medicine today. Surgery, by essence, is a field that requires the ability to bounce back from difficult situations. Surgical training tests an individual's ability to tolerate grueling work hours, intense physical and emotional stress, and maximum absorption and comprehension of vast amounts of medical and surgical knowledge. There is no doubt that every surgical resident has at some point felt the elation and despair of patient care.

There are three key principles or characteristics of resilient people that Diane Coutu puts forth in a poignant Harvard Business Review article entitled *How Resilience Works*—face down reality, search for meaning, and continually improvise. Resilient people possessed three defining characteristics. They coolly accept the harsh realities facing them. They find meaning in terrible times. And they have an uncanny ability to improvise.

Optimism and resilience are different. Blind optimism can distort perception of reality and cause problems. Resilient leaders do not slip into denial to cope with hardship. Prepare to act in ways that enables one to endure—train to survive before the fact. So, face down reality.

When complications occur or things go bad, do not cry victim. Find meaning in the suffering for all members of the team and plan for a better future. Use the hardship as motivation but do not let it weaken you. For examples, get angry about major surgical complications but use them as an opportunity to improve.

When disaster hits, be inventive—even if that means letting one's inner child out in a world that is dominated by gravity and urgency. Individuals should make the most of what they have and imagine possibilities others do not see. So, continually improvise.

7.1.4   Summary

Surgical residency is a privilege and honor. Patients welcome surgeons into the most intimate moments and aspects of their lives. With this honor, there comes significant responsibility to respect and value the day-to-day interactions needed to provide quality surgical care. The core of becoming a successful surgeon starts within oneself. The need to foster an environment conducive to effective teamwork, communication, and leadership is paramount to the performance of surgical teams. Continual self reflection and improvement is key to making this work. It is never too early to start.

Suggested Reading

Cameron KS, et al. Competing values leadership. Cheltenham: Edward Elgar Publishing; 2014.
Coutu DL. How resilience works. Harv Bus Rev. 2002;80(5):46–56.
Kouzes J, Barry P. The leadership challenge: how to make extraordinary things happen. Atlanta: Better World Books; 2012.
Staub R. Heart of leadership. Provo: Executive Excellence Publishing; 2000.

Chapter 8
Learning Surgery as a Student

Michael J. Englesbe and Patrick Underwood

Abstract Surgery is a uniquely rewarding career. High-performance on student surgery rotations is important for students who desire to become surgeons. Students must remain self-critical and thoughtful regarding their career choice, analyze the values and styles of surgical trainees and faculty on rotation. Maintain a rigorous schedule of didactic learning and reading while on rotation, never show up for the operating room unprepared. Great students have situational awareness, seek advice from junior house officers regarding ways to add value to patient care on the surgery rotation. Becoming a successful surgeon mandates a life of learning and self critical reflection. These habits begin as a medical student on the surgery service.

8.1 The Goal: Develop into a "Mature" Surgical Residency Applicant

It is not critical to decide on a post-medical school specialty prior to August of the fourth year of medical school. Many extraordinary students struggle with their career choice and delay a final decision until this late time. Considering the gravity of the decision, no good mentor would criticize a student for being thoughtful about it.

Surgical residency programs seek a "mature applicant." This label refers to students who have an in-depth understanding of surgery and how they plan to make an impact on healthcare. Presenting as a "mature applicant" has little to do with medical knowledge and more to do with non-clinical, professional and personal development goals. Developing into a "mature applicant" requires broad mentorship from accomplished surgeons and in-depth exposure to the field. Students who come from medical schools with an extensive academic surgical pedigree have a significant

M.J. Englesbe (✉)
Transplantation Surgery, University of Michigan Health Systems, Ann Arbor, MI, USA
e-mail: englesbe@med.umich.edu

P. Underwood
University of Florida, Gainesville, FL, USA
e-mail: underwood@surgery.ufl.edu

© Springer International Publishing Switzerland 2017   51
M.J. Englesbe, M.O. Meyers (eds.), *A How To Guide For Medical Students*,
Success in Academic Surgery, DOI 10.1007/978-3-319-42897-0_8

advantage and usually present themselves as "mature" residency applicants. There are approximately 20 schools that fulfill this category. Students who do not attend one of these schools should carefully pursue experiences that augment exposure to academic surgery and seek mentorship from more academic surgeons. Skills of "mature" residency applicants develop during career conversations with mentors, surgery rotations, away rotations, and through attending academic and professional meetings.

8.1.1 Do I Need to Know "Surgery" Before My Surgery Rotation?

8.1.1.1 Prior to Entering Medical School

Approximately one out of three surgeons knew surgery was going to be their career path prior to entering medical school. Even for these students, it is mandatory to focus on a broad array of experiences that will inform personal and career development. Surgery is not a core topic within pre-medical education and it is challenging to learn surgery prior to entering medical school. More importantly, it is not important to learn. For the motivated and focused pre-medical student, research and employment in surgery offer meaningful opportunity. Working in a surgical lab or in the operating room as an anesthesia technician are common jobs obtained by pre-medical students interested in surgery. These jobs offer unique opportunities for early exposure to a career in surgery and inform an application to medical school.

8.1.1.2 Should I Do a Lot of Shadowing as a Pre-clinical Student?

Clinical shadowing in the pre-clinical years of medical school informs career decision-making. This is particularly relevant in sub-specialty surgical fields, such as urology or vascular surgery. It is possible to go through the required clinical clerkship in surgery without seeing many exciting and impactful surgical fields. Clinical shadowing increases exposure to faculty and bolsters fund of knowledge. As an early medical student, clinical shadowing can reenergize students and provide an exhilarating break from the classroom.

Clinical shadowing should not impede foundational learning. There is plenty of time to rotate on surgical services later in the curriculum rather than miss important opportunities to build medical knowledge. One half day a month is a good amount of shadowing.

8.1.2   Developing the Non-clinical Skills of Surgery

Students who did not perceive themselves as "fitting" the stereotype of a surgeon frequently struggle with their career decision. Underlying this stereotype are specific skills and personality traits that are useful in a surgical career. Students who do not have these skills may struggle in surgery as a medical student and potentially in their career as a surgeon. Good mentors will help students explore their strengths and weaknesses and should frankly advise them whether they think they will be happy with a career in surgery. Nonclinical skills that exceptional surgeons possess include:

1. Decisiveness: surgeons have to make important decisions in a setting of limited information.
2. Resilience: patients will have poor outcomes related to surgeon performance and decision-making. Great surgeons are always self-critical but remain emotionally resilient in difficult situations.
3. Collaboration: surgery is a team sport. Great surgeons enjoy opportunities to work within effective teams for optimal care. Surgical culture has changed in the last decade. Obnoxious and self-centered surgeons are rare among surgical trainees and young attending surgeons.
4. Engagement: surgeons are not "laid back." Surgeons deeply care and relish the opportunity to be responsible for the wellness of their patient.

These skills are more important than fund of knowledge or manual dexterity. As a medical student on the surgery rotation, remain observant of the behaviors and personality types of the surgical team. Remain reflective about "fit" within surgical culture and ask surgeons about these important issues. Medical school curricula focusing on leadership skills for self-directed learning help optimally prepare students for their surgery rotations.

8.1.3   Learning Surgery During the Core Surgery Clerkship

8.1.3.1   Performing on the Wards

The majority of medical students are assigned to a specific care team. This team can be large (our transplant service rounds with 20 people each morning), and it is critical to understand everyone's roles and responsibilities. The attending surgeon is responsible for all of the care of the patient, but he or she is not present during early morning rounds on most days. The team is lead by a "Chief" resident or surgical fellow. This individual is in their last year or two of clinical training in surgery and is responsible for the day-to-day care of all patients on the service. Middle-level residents on the team manage consultations, new admissions, and perform many of the surgical procedures. A team will frequently have several interns from many fields, including anesthesia. The intern's primary job is to manage the details of care such as placing orders, collecting clinical information, and writing notes. Many teams have nurse practitioners and physician assistants, pharmacists, and nutritionists. These individuals assure continuity and are experts in the normal protocols of care. They are a robust resource for educational content.

It is challenging for students to figure out how to add value to the care of patients within the fast-paced and complex process of inpatient surgical care. Great students have situational awareness; they know when to help and when to step back. The chief resident will round on all patients on the service with remarkable speed; it can be difficult to keep up. Junior members of the care team are able to provide advice on how to add value to morning rounds. Students will be responsible for pre-rounding and reporting data, dressing changes, and other care tasks during morning rounds. Coordination with the other students, physician extenders, and interns will facilitate seamless progress through morning rounds.

Teamwork, enthusiasm, and engagement are the hallmarks of the exceptional medical student. Know the details of care for every patient on the service. Always be willing to help in any task that will facilitate patient care and efficiency. Always be early and prepared for morning rounds. Working hard and adding value to the care of patients on a busy but effective surgical service can be among the most rewarding experiences of medical school. Conversely, difficult personalities coupled with fatigue and sick patients foster an environment that is deleterious to patient care and learning. Extraordinary students transcend challenging team dynamics by focusing on patient-centered care and learning. Much can be learned when a team is not functioning well; discuss these situations with mentors and learn from them. Struggles with fellow students must be handled discretely and largely ignored unless they are affecting patient care.

8.1.3.2   Learning from Every Patient

The most effective way to build foundational surgical knowledge and study for examinations is to learn from every patient. There are many hours of downtime between cases and while awaiting rounds. Successful students fill this time with learning. Every patient offers a wealth of opportunities to review anatomy, physiology, and other key topics. Exceptional students ask themselves "why" specific management decisions or clinical outcomes occurred. These students have the discipline to question accepted mechanisms of disease and surgical tradition and strive to learn evidence-based practices. Beginning this discovery process with a specific patient provides context and structure to learning. Read about patients every night in preparation to provide exceptional care tomorrow.

8.1.3.3 Preparation for the Operating Room

Students must come to the operating room prepared. If appropriate, introduce yourself to the patient and his/her family and explain the role of a medical student on the surgical team. Ask the patient about their disease, its effect on their life, and what they hope the surgery will achieve. Follow the patient closely throughout their entire hospital course. Have the discipline to repeatedly ask why specific decisions were made and to fill in knowledge gaps with inquiry.

Attending surgeons and house officers assess students for fund of knowledge and clinical judgment during surgery. Students must have an in-depth understanding of the clinical details of the patient and the disease process being addressed with the intended surgery. Even in emergency surgical care, there is usually time for a student to pause and do some reading. Vast resources are available to inform clinical knowledge, operative anatomy, and technical challenges of the procedure.

8.1.3.4 Preparing for the Oral Examination

The oral examination has a long history within surgery. Surgeons consider it the ultimate test of competency. Upon completion of residency training, surgical specialties administer an oral examination. Many surgical residency programs have trainees take annual oral examinations. Most medical student surgery clerkships require students to pass an oral examination. Few events in medical school cause more anxiety than this examination.

The cornerstone of student clinical competency in this examination is organization. Deep clinical knowledge of the topics covered on this examination must be coupled with an organized assessment of a surgically ill patient. A simple template that is applicable to surgical patients (trauma patient assessment follows a different model) must be practiced (Fig. 8.1). This template is relevant not only for this examination but throughout clinical practice. It assures comprehensive assessment and management of a sick patient. The authors use this template every day when assessing a severely ill patient.

8.1.3.5 Studying for the Written Exam

Most medical students do well during the subjective assessments of performance on the clinical rotation. As a result, the majority of the variance among medical student grades results from examinations. The "SHELF" examination is a surgery subject examination for medical students provided by the National Board of Medical Examiners. Most medical schools use this as a "final" exam. The content of the examination is comprehensive; it is impossible to study all that will be on the test. Study materials that provide a robust number of questions are effective.

Fig. 8.1 Organizational template for patient assessment. "Are they sick or not" means assess vitals/ ABCs. In adults, if the blood pressure is less than 100 or heart rate over 100, intervention is necessary prior to continuing with the next step

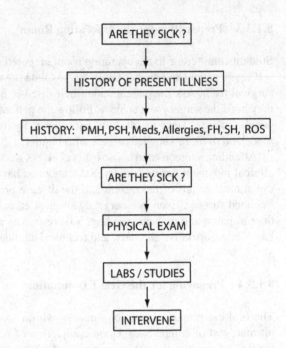

Study questions facilitate goal directed studying; wrong answers motivate learning and fill gaps in knowledge. Studying for this examination must start at the beginning of the clerkship.

8.1.4   Post Clerkship Surgical Education

8.1.4.1   Sub-internships

Sub-internships occur in the first few months of the final year of medical school. These clinical rotations solidify residency selection. Performance on these rotations is used for faculty letters of recommendation. Strategic timing and exposure to key personnel is important when scheduling these rotations.

Great surgical sub-interns blend seamlessly into the team and add value at every turn. It is mandatory that a sub-intern collaborates with and mentors junior medical students who are also on the rotation. Overly enthusiastic sub-interns may demonstrate their inability to work within the team by the way they treat the other medical students. This is the single most common event that deleteriously affects a high-performing medical student's reputation. Complex dynamics among students rotating on the same service can be challenging; frank and discrete discussions with a trusted surgical house officer can help manage these difficult situations. Avoid mentioning these occurrences to faculty unless the situation is affecting patient care.

Surgical residents expect sub-interns to work hard. Students must demonstrate toughness. Come in early, leave late, and always be prepared. It is rare that medical students are given important responsibilities for patient care; if this happens, remain conservative and humble. Never hesitate to ask for assistance or help. Asking for help is a sign of commitment to exceptional patient care and is not a sign of weakness.

Surgical sub-interns must remain self-critical about their clinical performance. Great surgeons blame themselves first and use clinical challenges as opportunities for self-improvement. Students frequently struggle with the pace and intensity of the sub-internship. This is normal and will be mastered with time. Remain thoughtful regarding career decisions. If a sub-intern finds the hours overwhelming or is not excited about the proposition of becoming a surgical house-officer, re-consider career choices.

8.1.4.2 Extramural Rotations

Rotating at an institution where you have interest in matching has significant advantages and disadvantages. The advantages of these rotations include:

1. Away rotations provide audition opportunities. This is important for students from smaller and lower "pedigree" medical schools.
2. Away rotations inform match choices. If you have strong interest in a specific program, rotate there to confirm interest.
3. Away rotations develop students into more mature applicants. Exposure outside of the home institution broadens a student's personal narrative regarding career plans.

The disadvantages include:

1. Logistical challenges – frequently medical school schedules do not overlap.
2. Performing on a surgical sub-internship in an unfamiliar city can be challenging.
3. Different medical schools have different expectations of fourth year medical students; it takes time to settle into the flow of care at a new institution.

Away rotations are thought to be particularly important in orthopedic, vascular, and cardiothoracic surgery but remain less critical in general surgery.

8.1.4.3 Other Clinical Rotations That Inform Clinical Development

Graduate medical education is rigorous and focused. Surgical training affords minimal elective opportunities. There is ample time to learn surgery during surgical residency; take opportunities to develop diverse foundational clinical knowledge. All students going into a surgical field should rotate on an anesthesia service.

In addition, suggested clinical rotations, stratified by specialty, are detailed in the table below.

General	Vascular	Plastics	Orthopedics	Cardiothoracics	Urology
Gastroenterology	Cardiology	Vascular surgery	Rheumatology	Cardiology	Nephrology
Nephrology	Interventional radiology	Dermatology	Plastic surgery	Pulmonology	Gastroenterology
Urology	Nephrology	Oral-Max-Face surgery	Physical-med rehabilitation	Nephrology	Radiation oncology
Neurosurgery	Plastic surgery	Surgical oncology	Trauma surgery	Geriatrics	Geriatrics
Medical oncology	Geriatrics	Orthopedic surgery	Radiology	Medical oncology	Ob-Gyn

8.1.4.4   Surgery Boot Camps

Some medical schools offer surgical "boot camps" prior to graduation. Keeping senior medical students engaged in the curriculum is challenging in the final months of medical school. These "boot camp" rotations work well when placed a month or two prior to graduation. The goal of these courses is to prepare students for surgical residency "Day One". These rotations offer a pragmatic and fun opportunity to hone clinical judgment and technical skills. The curriculum should include a mock-paging program, surgical anatomy, discussions on house officer wellness, and opportunities to hone procedure-based skills through simulation. Students report that the boot camp rotations are extremely valuable in preparing them for surgical internship.

8.1.5   Summary

Surgery is a uniquely rewarding and challenging career. For future surgeons, the goals of medical school surgery education are to provide foundational knowledge and empower students to become mature residency applicants with a well-formed vision of how they will impact healthcare. Becoming a successful surgeon mandates a life of learning and self-critical reflection. These habits begin to form as a medical student rotating on the surgical services. Students should pay attention to the intangible skills that surgeons possess such as the ability to work in teams, the desire to lead, and the ability to remain enthusiastic, despite the rigors of surgical care. Developing these skills as a student is an important beginning to a young surgeon's career.

Chapter 9
The Fourth Year of Medical School for the Surgery Student

David T. Hughes

Abstract The fourth year of medical school is an exciting time for students as it is the culmination of medical school and the time when students prepare for residency. This chapter will focus on the preparation and process of making the year a successful capstone for medical school and a solid foundation for surgical residency.

9.1   Introduction

The fourth year of medical school is an exciting time for students as it is the culmination of medical school and the time when students prepare for residency. These priorities should be complementary rather than competing, and students should keep both in mind as they formulate their rotation schedules, decide whether to do away rotations and where, identify faculty mentors to ask for letters of recommendation, and prepare for the rigors and logistics of being a surgical resident. This chapter will focus on the preparation and process of making the year a successful capstone for medical school and a solid foundation for surgical residency.

9.2   M4 Rotation Scheduling

Scheduling for the fourth year of medical school typically begins in the spring of the M3 year when students have completed most of the M3 clinical clerkships and have often chosen a career specialty. The logistics of creating an M4 rotation schedule depend on a number of factors, some of which are dictated by the medical school, some by residency application deadlines, and some by the student's clinical and academic interests. For students who are undecided, the beginning of the M4 year allows for continued exploration of specialties and sub-specialties to solidify decisions about career choices. In addition to rotations, the M4 year should include

D.T. Hughes (✉)
University of Michigan, Ann Arbor, MI, USA
e-mail: davhughe@med.umich.edu

© Springer International Publishing Switzerland 2017
M.J. Englesbe, M.O. Meyers (eds.), *A How To Guide For Medical Students,*
Success in Academic Surgery, DOI 10.1007/978-3-319-42897-0_9

completion of Step 2 of the boards, scheduled away rotations, time for residency interviews, and time for vacation (Fig. 9.1).

When planning their M4 schedule, students should attempt to place their most preferable rotations towards the beginning of the year, especially in cases where sub-internship (sub-I) or specialty rotations may allow them to come to a final decision about career specialty. Most medical schools use a lottery system in allocating rotations; surgical subspecialties such as orthopedics, plastic surgery, and otolaryngology often fill quickly. M3 students should seek faculty and resident mentors who can provide guidance about specialty and rotation choices for the M4 year. Mentors in the student's specialty of choice can also discuss the value of away rotations in the residency application process, as well as possible locations for these away rotations (discussed further below).

Medical schools typically require one or two sub-I rotations, often in medicine, surgery, or the student's future specialty. For students interested in surgery, these occur on surgical services in the student's sub-specialty of choice. Sub-I's serve many purposes: they solidify or clarify a student's specialty of choice, allow increasing clinical responsibility appropriate for senior medical students, provide education on the perioperative management of patients, prepare students for the demands of internship, and facilitate the identification of faculty mentors who can provide career counseling and letters of recommendation. Because the residency application process begins in September of the M4 year, students experience the greatest benefits by completing sub-I rotations at the beginning of the academic year.

Required rotations are less time-dependent should be scheduled after obtaining sub-I rotations; these may include critical care, medical specialties (e.g., cardiology or nephrology), emergency medicine, neurology, radiology, and outpatient care.

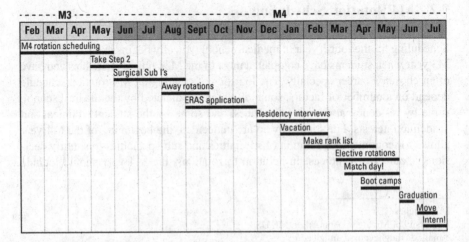

Fig. 9.1 Traditional timeline for late M3 and the M4 year

Students should avoid the "pre-residency syndrome" (thinking only of preparation for residency during the M4 year) and not lose sight of the educational opportunities that the final year of medical school provides. When surgical residents and faculty are asked which rotations during the M4 year were the most valuable throughout their careers, most rank medical specialties relevant to their surgical specialty at the top of the list. Typical non-surgical rotations relevant to surgical specialties, such as radiology, cardiology, nephrology, and pulmonology, are discussed in the chapter entitled "Learning surgery as a student."

Most medical schools allow students to dedicate a month, typically December or January, to residency interviews. Students should consider scheduling either vacation time or elective rotations with a lighter workload during interview season (November to January) to allow for increased flexibility in scheduling interviews outside of the "interview month." One month is usually enough time to allow for eight interviews; students attending more than eight may find it helpful to increase the available time to 2 months.

After interview season, students should continue to take advantage of elective rotations to broaden their clinical exposure outside their specialty of choice. Each student is responsible for creating a valuable educational experience most applicable to his/her individual interests and future career plans. Opportunities abound for fourth year students to increase levels of clinical responsibility and gain experiences beyond the surgical specialties seen during the third year surgery rotation. Students should seek out education about pathophysiology encountered in their specialty that requires consultation with another specialty. Learning radiology, revisiting anatomy and other basic science topics, and honing skills in critical care or complex patient management will prepare students for internship and practice. Many medical schools offer surgical residency prep courses (boot camps) during the last few months of the M4 year. These courses are well received because they provide relevant and timely clinical management knowledge and technical skills.

9.3 Away Rotations

Most students are limited to two away rotations due to requirements at their home medical school as well as the time constraints of the residency application process. Away rotations are often considered to serve two purposes: to provide the surgical student the opportunity to experience surgery at another institution and to "audition" for a surgical residency position at that institution. Several studies have evaluated the effect of away rotations on the residency match process and concluded that away rotations do not appear to influence how residency programs rank students (Vogt et al. 2000; Tzarnas and Fessenden 2002; Fabri et al. 1995). Despite this, some specialties, particularly orthopedics and plastic surgery, continue to emphasize the importance of away rotations for a successful match. Due to conflicting views on the value of audition rotations, students should focus instead on evaluating how well the institution suits them, asking such questions as:

- Is this the kind of place that provides what I need for residency?
- Do I fit in with the other residents, the faculty and the staff?
- Is the geographic location right for me and/or my family?

Away rotations also provide the visiting student context to practices learned at their home institutions and insight into the differing structures and qualities of surgical residency programs and health systems. Students who are interested in matching at the surgical residency program they are visiting should be vocal about this and try to meet with the program director during their rotation to make their interest known as well as to learn more about the program. After completing an away rotation, students can set themselves apart by sending thank you notes to their primary faculty contact, the program director (if they met with him or her), and the residents they worked with the most during the rotation.

The benefits of away rotations must be weighed against the disadvantages. The costs of travel and accommodations in another city can add up quickly and exceed what some students can afford, especially considering the impending costs of residency interviews. Being away from the home institution can interfere with communication and the ability to meet with faculty from surgical sub-I rotations regarding letters of recommendations. Scheduling away rotations can also be logistically challenging due to the differing rotation time periods at other institutions, requiring close communication with the registrar's office at both institutions.

Overall, the decision to do an away rotation should come down to the student's interest in an institution's residency program as it is an opportunity for deeper insight into a program than can be determined from just one interview day.

9.4   Getting Letters of Recommendation

Students need three or four letters of recommendation for the ERAS application. For surgical residencies, most, if not all, of the letters should be authored by surgeons, either within or outside the specialty of choice. Letters from faculty outside the surgical specialties can be valuable as long as these letter writers know the student well and speak to qualities about which they are uniquely knowledgeable due to their interactions with the student. Students who are applying to more than one specialty might consider using a different combination of letters for each specialty; the ERAS application allows for this.

Students should solicit letters from faculty as early as possible, but no later than a month in advance of the deadline, to ensure they have plenty of time to complete the letters prior to the ERAS release to programs in mid-September. Asking for letters of recommendation is done in person or via email and should not be an onerous prospect for students because faculty are expecting these requests. Meeting with each letter writer in person to talk about career interests, personal experiences, and possible residency programs also offers an ideal time for mentoring and career counseling beyond just what is needed for the letter of recommendation. Once the faculty member has agreed to write a letter, the student should provide him/her an updated curriculum vitae (CV) as the letter writer may wish to reference accomplishments listed in the CV. Having a copy of the personal statement may also help the faculty to write a more distinctive and individualized letter; the faculty may also give feedback about the content and quality of the student's personal statement. Students should waive their rights to see the letters of recommendation and be sure to provide the ERAS application number to letter writers to allow them to upload letters to the ERAS site. It should be noted that this process differs for students applying to urology, ophthalmology, or who have a military obligation. Appropriate career counseling should be sought out by students applying to these specialties.

Determining which faculty to ask for a letter of recommendation depends on a student's rotation experience, the personalities of both the faculty and student, and the overall theme the student wants portrayed in the residency application. The most important and valuable letter comes from a faculty member who knows the student on a personal level and who can discuss the student's clinical performance, communication abilities, knowledge base, technical skills, personality traits, and future plans, having directly observed the student in a multitude of settings including clinic, the operating room, the wards, and in other professional venues. A mediocre letter of recommendation discusses a student in broad terms without specific examples and often only reiterates the information in the CV. A great letter of recommendation talks about the student in specifics, gives examples of his/her performance based on personal interactions or observations, talks about the student's personality and demeanor, and tells stories or anecdotes about how the student performs. Students should request letters from faculty who will portray their unique and outstanding characteristics in a straightforward and detailed manner. These are usually the two or three faculty members students have spent the most time with, whether during M3 and M4 surgery rotations, on a research lab/project, or as part of an academic or global health project.

Many institutions have the Chair or Chief of Surgery write a letter for any student applying to their specialty. This letter holds weight as long as the letter writer knows the student well enough to discuss the student in specifics. Setting up a brief meeting with the Chair or Chief of Surgery is highly recommended and goes a long way in providing the letter writer with specifics about a student's interests, qualities, and personal history which will lead to a higher quality letter.

9.5 Interviews and Vacation Time

During the M4 year, students will spend about 25 % of their time either on residency interviews or vacation. Interviews are the most important part of the M4 year with respect to obtaining a residency position. Students typically interview at anywhere between 5 and 20 programs depending on the quality of their application, the competiveness of their specialty of choice, personal restrictions (such as geography or couples matching), and desire to interview. Because each program visit typically includes an evening gathering with the residents followed by a full day of speeches, interviews and tours, as well as travel time on both ends, most visits require 2 days. Students who accept ten or more interviews may find that scheduling difficulties, cost, and stress are all magnified. Having more than 1 month to dedicate to interviews during interview season (typically from November to January) will lessen these headaches, but will often require scheduling non-clinical rotations or vacation time during interview season.

In deciding how many interviews to attend, students may wish to consider the following questions:

- How competitive am I compared to other students?
- How competitive is the specialty?
- What are the odds of matching in that specialty relative to the number of interviews attended?
- How much do I want to spend?

The National Resident Matching Program (NRMP) releases the match data yearly, which can help students understand the overall competitiveness of both their specialty of choice and their own application (http://www.nrmp.org/match-data/main-residency-match-data/). The number of programs a student ranks in the NRMP is directly proportional to likelihood of a successful match. An interview at a program is a requirement for the program to rank a student. Students should interview at enough programs to allow them to be ranked by 8–12 programs. Presuming that students decide not to include a few of the programs at which they interviewed on their match list, a reasonable target number of interviews should be 8–14, adjusted as needed depending on competitiveness.

Containing costs during the interview season is often desirable but difficult to achieve due to additive transportation and accommodation expenses. Some programs offer hosting at their institution or help with connecting fellow interviewing students to share a hotel room. Students should inquire about this when scheduling the interview. Grouping interviews in geographic proximity allows for reduced transportation costs, although is not always feasible due to availability of interview dates.

The M4 year is not all work and no play. Most programs take a break from interviews over the holiday season in late December and early January, giving students a chance to relax and spend time with friends and family. Medical school graduation is typically in the late spring, which allows time for a long vacation before the start of residency. Students should be sure to take care of any paperwork requirements for starting residency and make arrangements for the move well in advance of the traditional July 1st start date and should anticipate an orientation 1–2 weeks prior to starting intern year.

9.6 Residency Preparation Courses ("Boot Camps")

During the final months of medical school, most students are focused on preparing to start their internship in July. To aid in that goal, many medical schools include residency preparation courses, also known as boot camps, as an elective (or required) rotation after interview season. The content and length of these courses vary between institutions; however, the American College of Surgeons, the Association of Program Directors in Surgery, and the Association of Surgical Education are in the midst of a joint effort to develop a standardized national curriculum for preparation for surgical residency (https://www.facs.org/education/program/resident-prep). This curriculum is available to all medical schools and includes such content areas as: first response to unstable patient, emergency procedures, management of electrolyte abnormalities, management of perioperative conditions, radiograph interpretation, operative anatomy, responding to pages from nurses, handoffs, dealing with difficult patients, communication, and informed consent. Some institutions notify residency program directors whether incoming students have completed a residency prep course, as these students may require a lower level of initial supervision. The surgical boot camp will likely soon become a standard experience during the final year of medical school for students heading into surgical residency.

9.7 Conclusion

Fourth year medical students should make the most of abundant opportunities for growth as they develop enhanced clinical skills with increasing responsibility and the maturity necessary for success as a future surgeon. Putting thought into and seeking mentorship to navigate the residency application process is worthwhile as the match will determine not only their future specialty, but also the course of their professional identity. Students should gear up for an eventful year and enjoy the journey.

References

American College of Surgeons/Association of Program Directors in Surgery/Association for Surgical Education Resident Prep Curriculum: https://www.facs.org/education/program/resident-prep

Fabri PJ, Powell DL, Cupps NB. Is there value in audition extramurals? Am J Surg. 1995;169:338–40.

National Resident Matching Program (NRMP) Main Residency Match Data: http://www.nrmp.org/match-data/main-residency-match-data/

Tzarnas CD, Fessenden J. Audition electives during the surgical residency and selection for post-residency fellowship positions. Curr Surg. 2002;59:412–5.

Vogt HB, Thanel FH, Hearns VL. The audition elective and its relation to success in the National Resident Matching Program. Teach Learn Med. 2000;12:78–80.

Chapter 10
Developing a Research Portfolio as a Medical Student

Shannon L. Cramm, Benjamin Levi, and Dorry Segev

Stay far from timid, Only make moves when your heart's in it,
And live the phrase: 'The sky's the limit.' (Notorious B.I.G).

Abstract Research drives medicine forward: The ability to formulate and answer scientific questions about the human body, disease, medicine, and healthcare delivery allows physicians to improve patient care. Thus, engaging in research is a natural step for students who have committed their professional lives to the health of others. This chapter will discuss why research experience is important for medical students, the types of research in medicine, and how students can be successful in building their research portfolio during medical school. This chapter examines ways to improve each step of the process: from deciding on a mentor and specialty, to completing a research project, to packaging a research portfolio in a curriculum vita.

10.1 Why Do Research as a Medical Student?

Research drives medicine forward. Whether it's the development of novel agents for anesthesia or the discovery of the role *H. pylori* plays in the pathogenesis of gastritis, the ability to formulate and answer scientific questions about the human body, disease, medicine, and healthcare delivery allows physicians to improve patient

S.L. Cramm • B. Levi
University of Michigan, Ann Arbor, MI, USA
e-mail: slcramm@med.umich.edu; blevi@med.umich.edu

D. Segev (✉)
Johns Hopkins School of Medicine, Baltimore, MD, USA
e-mail: dorry@jhmi.edu

© Springer International Publishing Switzerland 2017
M.J. Englesbe, M.O. Meyers (eds.), *A How To Guide For Medical Students,*
Success in Academic Surgery, DOI 10.1007/978-3-319-42897-0_10

care. Thus, engaging in research is a natural step for students who have committed their professional lives to the health of others. The discovery of heparin, insulin, ether anesthesia, and the Sphincter of Oddi are just some of the advances through which research has shaped the field of surgery; all were medical student discoveries (Stringer and Ahmadi 2009). A medical student is at the very impetus of a lifelong career and performing research at this early stage has substantial value – not the least of which is innovating the field so that physicians are better equipped to care for patients.

The idea of conducting meaningful research may seem overwhelming to a student at the beginning of their medical training, especially considering they likely have not received any formal training in this area. For students interested in a career in an academic setting, starting research projects while in medical school allows them to develop essential skills under the guidance of medical school faculty that will serve them in their future careers: The ability to formulate scientific questions, design appropriate studies, write successful grants, analyze results, trouble shoot challenges, and present the findings through presentations will serve students throughout their career.

For those students who are interested in community or private practice, research during medical school allows them to develop other important transferable skills including critical thinking, problem solving, and written and oral communication skills. Honing these abilities will help students to become better clinicians, leaders, and team members regardless of the setting in which they ultimately decide to work. Experience with research will also improve students' ability to read and interpret scientific literature, which is an essential for any practicing clinician. Indeed, with the ever-growing body of knowledge in medicine, the ability to think critically, problem solve, and acquire new knowledge is integral to the future physician.

Beyond developing a research skillset, engaging in research in medical school gives students a unique opportunity to gain a better understanding of a particular specialty that they are interested in exploring as a future career. This occurs (1) by developing an understanding of current research and direction of the field and (2) through networking with current professionals. Research offers multiple opportunities for these experiences. For instance, in preparing for a research proposal or a manuscript, a student will complete in-depth literature reviews and become familiar with the body of work relevant to their project. In the process of working with a research group, students may have the opportunity to attend group meetings to learn about other projects and meet professionals working in the field. These research mentors – including both faculty and residents – provide an invaluable insight into the field in which they practice.

In publicizing and publishing their work, students may attend regional, national, or international research conferences and academic meetings. In these settings, students will be exposed to the breadth of research in their particular field. They will also have the opportunity to meet and network with leaders in the field from other institutions whom students otherwise may not have the opportunity to meet. Many of these meetings have travel funding and activities designed specifically for trainees, of which students should take full advantage. Furthermore, this deeper understanding of their future field will help students to be more successful in their clinical rotations and ultimately in their residency interviews.

Additionally, the clinicians, trainees, and scientists with whom students meet and work during the research experiences can become important mentors through a student's time in medical school, residency, and career. Having knowledgeable and invested mentorship is a critical element in a student's career success. By participating in research with the right mentor (see section "What Makes a Good Mentor"), students have a unique opportunity to work one-on-one over long periods of time with a dedicated physician-scientist in their future specialty. Unlike the interactions students have with faculty in lectures and on the wards, which are often limited by length of duration, the number of students, and clinical duties, the longer-term and more in-depth interaction that research projects require helps to foster deeper connections for meaningful mentorship.

All of the above benefits of research for medical students – a commitment to innovation, developing transferable skills, establishing an understanding of the field, and fostering mentoring relationships – translate into the final benefit: enhancing a student's application to residency. This benefit is intentionally listed last. While this is often the focal point of many medical students as they consider pursuing a research project, it is important to understand that research enhances an application to residency because of the aforementioned benefits, and a student should not pursue a research opportunity without the utmost commitment to their project, their research mentors, and the development of their research skills.

Research experience is undeniably an essential part of a strong residency application in academic surgery – one study found that 73 % of applicants in 2014–2015 at 33 surgery programs had at least one publication, and another reported that 76.8 % of top 20-ranked applicants to 22 general surgery programs had research experience (Dort et al. 2015; Stain et al. 2013). This number is even higher for highly competitive surgical programs and subspecialties, often more than 90 % of applicants (Tchantchaleishvili et al. 2013). Quality research experiences in which a student acquires skills and demonstrates productivity are key to distinguish students. Thus the rest of this chapter will discuss strategies for medical students to successfully and purposefully begin creating their research portfolios while in medical school.

Summary
- Engaging in research is valuable because new medical observations and discoveries improve our ability to care for patients and populations.
- Students interested in an academic career should start research in medical school because it is a skillset that takes time to develop.
- Research as a medical student has substantial benefits for students pursuing careers in community practice. The skills research fosters such as problem solving and critical thinking are essential to being an effective physician.
- Research allows students to explore in depth a field in which they may want to specialize.

- Research allows students to develop meaningful resident and faculty mentorship in a particular field.
- Research enhances a student's application to residency.

10.2 Choosing a Research Area

The first step for a student interested in developing a research portfolio is to decide what type of research they are interested in doing, specifically (1) what specialty and (2) type of research.

10.2.1 Specialty

In the first year of medical school when a student may be considering various career paths, the decision of what specialty to start research in may seem overwhelming. However, the specialty in which a student does research is much less important than whether the student does research at all. A student should choose a field in which they are interested, but should not delay starting to develop their research skills until they have committed to a field. Many students do not decide on a particular specialty until their late third or early fourth years. Nor should they feel limited to applying to a field in which they've done research come fourth year. Choosing a topic of research applicable to multiple specialties improves the chances their research will be applicable to their future specialty.

However, a student interested in highly competitive specialties may benefit during residency applications by demonstrating a longitudinal interest, developing mentors early, and publishing in that particular field. Highly competitive surgical specialties include plastic surgery, orthopaedic surgery, neurosurgery, urology, and otolaryngology. Thus, if a student feels they may be interested in these or other highly competitive specialties, it would be wise to use research in the first years of medical school as an avenue to explore that field as a possible career as well as begin developing a field-specific research portfolio. If a student is interested in several competitive specialties, they should choose projects and mentors based on their level of interest as well the type of research projects and mentors available, which will be described in later sections.

10.2.2 Types of Medical Research

Before diving into the process of finding a research mentor in the specialty a student has selected, it is important to have a basic understanding of the various types of research. This will allow the student to seek projects that best suit their career goals, interests, and schedule. Broadly, research can be divided into basic medical and clinical research. In this section, these areas as well as subsets will be briefly described. Special areas of medical education research and global health research will also be highlighted.

10.2.3   Basic Medical Research

Medical research			
Basic medical research		Clinical research	
Theoretical	Applied	Interventional	Observational
Method	Animal study	Clinical trials (Phases 0–1)	Cohort study
Development	Cell study	Cohort study	Case control
	Genetic study		Registry study
	Biochemistry		Case series
	Material		Case report
	Development		
	Translational		
	Biomedical engineering		

Basic medical research is also often referred to as basic science, experimental, bench, or wet lab research. It includes a wide variety of animal, cellular, histological, genetic, biochemical, and physiologic studies on the properties of healthy and diseased systems, pathogens themselves, and treatments. Basic medical research also includes the development and improvement of analytical procedures, imaging methods, gene sequencing, and biometric procedures. Basic medical research generally includes experiments where the investigator directly alters an independent variable and the effects on dependent variable(s) are measured.

Examples of basic medical science projects in surgery include:

1. To understand how a lymph node excision changes the lymphatic flow and to evaluate the ability of lymphatic isolation to impair the immunologic response to transplanted allogeneic skin in a mouse model.
    Agarwal S, Loder S, Wood S, et al. Engendering allograft ignorance in a mouse model of allogeneic skin transplantation to the distal hind limb. Ann Surg. 2015;261(3):611–618.
2. To investigate the role of aldose reductase in hepatic ischemia-reperfusion injury and explore the underlying mechanisms in both human and rat models
    Li CX, Ng KT, Shao Y, et al. The inhibition of aldose reductase attenuates hepatic ischemia-reperfusion injury through reducing inflammatory response. Ann Surg. 2014;260(2):317–328.

From a learning perspective, students who participate in basic medical research may learn a wide variety of "wet lab" techniques specific to their project. For example, students may learn how to culture bacteria, human cells, or tissue. They may learn how to do procedures to obtain samples from animal models. They may learn how to complete Western blots or polymerase chain reactions. The types of skills they learn will be determined by the specific experiments being conducted in their project and lab. Students may also have the opportunity to learn how to perform statistical analysis.

Basic medical science is the foundation of our understanding of the science of medicine and is often a first step in medical innovation and discovery that ultimately translates into helping patients. It is a very rewarding process and depending on the area of study, will likely serve to augment a student's understanding of the basic science areas they are learning in the classroom, such as histology, physiology, genetics, or biochemistry. Students who participate in basic medical research will gain an in-depth understanding of the mechanisms relating to the organ system, disease process, or treatment being studied.

Notably, basic medical research projects are often resource and time intensive. This is something students should address with mentors as they begin a project. Students should ensure they have the proper oversight, materials, and direction in order to complete scientifically sound experiments that add meaningful information to the larger scientific project. As with any research endeavor, it is essential students have a clearly defined role within the project with mutually agreed upon endpoints and goals (see section "How to Maximize Productivity: Goal Setting").

10.2.4   Clinical Research

The hallmark of clinical research is that it involves the study of human volunteers to add to medical knowledge. This may be in the form of an Interventional Study, such as a clinical trial (Phase 0–4, as defined by the Food and Drug Administration) where new drugs, devices, or interventions are tested for safety and ultimately efficacy against a standard treatment, a placebo, or no intervention. Observational clinical research, also known as non-interventional clinical research or epidemiologic research, assesses outcomes of populations for whom investigators do not control interventions.

Clinical trials are generally very large undertakings that may be sponsored by a drug or device company or conducted independently. Given that they are always prospective, they often require long follow up times and are work intensive. While there are exceptions, these may not be ideal settings for medical students interested in developing research skills. However, for students with an appropriate, invested mentor and specific clinical project, interventional clinical research may be an appropriate project for dedicated research time, such as a yearlong research fellowship.

Observational clinical research, on the other hand, is often an excellent way for students to participate in research. Studies that are cross-sectional, retrospective, or analysis of present registry data are well geared towards students because the data is already available and there is no follow-up time required. Students can assist in these projects in a variety of ways including data collection (such as chart review), data analysis, literature review, and/or writing. However, much like basic medical research, the study design and analytical tools of observational research require advanced knowledge and training, so students should seek opportunities to work with mentors and groups with experience in these areas. Students who participate in observational clinical research may learn of clinically relevant information regarding the disease, population, and/or intervention they are studying. They may also learn about descriptive and analytic statistical methods as well as principles of epidemiology.

Examples of observational clinical research in surgery include:

1. To compare the risk of end-stage renal disease in living kidney donors to that of a healthy cohort of non-donors
   Muzaale AD, Massie AB, Wang MC, et al. Risk of end-stage renal disease following live kidney donation. JAMA. 2014;311(6):579–586.
2. To determine the relationship between oral antibiotic bowel preparation and surgical site infection in a national colectomy cohort
   Simianu VV, Strate LL, Billingham RP, et al. The Impact of Elective Colon Resection on Rates of Emergency Surgery for Diverticulitis. Ann Surg. 2016;263(1):123–129.

10.2.5   Special Topics

10.2.5.1   Medical Education Research

Medical education research is a broad area of research that includes the evaluation of the transfer and/or acquisition of knowledge, attitudes, and skills relevant to health and healthcare of learners, which can include students, trainees, health professionals, patients, or non-medical professional care providers (such as a spouse, etc.). Topics generally fall into one of the six professional core competencies as defined by the Accreditation Council of Graduate Medical Education (The General Surgery Milestone Project 2015):

1. Patient care
2. Medical knowledge
3. Practice-based learning and improvement
4. Interpersonal and communication skills
5. Systems-based practice
6. Professionalism.

This can be through interventional or observational methods. Medical education research is a form of clinical research where the interventions, observations, and outcomes are related in some way to understanding and improving medical education. These may be excellent opportunities for students to work closely with faculty interested in medical student and resident education. Medical education research can also be geared at the education of patients and may be ideal for students interested in implementing interventions to improve patient understanding of their health and healthcare.

Examples of medical education research include:

1. Flexibility in Duty Hour Requirements for Surgical Trainees (FIRST) Trial: to evaluate whether changing resident duty hour policies to permit greater flexibility in patient postoperative outcomes, resident education and resident well-being

   Bilimoria KY, Chung JW, Hedges LV, et al. Development of the Flexibility in Duty Hour Requirements for Surgical Trainees (FIRST) Trial Protocol: A National Cluster-Randomized Trial of Resident Duty Hour Policies. JAMA Surg. 2015:1–9.

2. To explore the development and transfer of knowledge of third-year preclinical students on problem-based learning (PBL) course with real patients

   Diemers AD, van de Wiel MW, Scherpbier AJ, Baarveld F, Dolmans DH. Diagnostic reasoning and underlying knowledge of students with preclinical patient contacts in PBL. Med Educ. 2015;49(12):1229–1238.

10.2.5.2 Global Health Research

The above research types and designs can also be completed in a global setting. Some medical schools may offer international elective opportunities for students to participate in research projects abroad with faculty and residents. There are also funding opportunities for students interested in taking dedicated time for research in global health (see section on "Funding Opportunities"). These are unique opportunities for students with particular interest in global health and can be a particularly rich learning experience given the additional considerations in conducting medical care and research in foreign countries. However, it is important that students consider the projects individually in regards to a student's own time availability and the skills they desire to learn from their research experience. As mentioned above, the most important thing in deciding on a research project is finding a quality opportunity to advance skills important to a given student. For some, projects in global health research may be perfectly suited. For others, it may be possible to engage in more meaningful work at their medical school or other academic institutions in order to better develop particular research skills.

Summary

In deciding what research project area to undertake, students should consider all aspects including specialty, research type, career goals, interests, and time commitment.

- Specialty:
  - Students should seek opportunities in fields that interest them, but should not wait to seek research opportunities until they have committed to a specialty.

- If interested in a highly competitive specialty, students should use early research projects as a way to investigate that possible career path and build their research portfolio in that area.

- Research Type:

  - Basic Medical Research: Describes a wide variety of experimental research to advance our understanding of the basic science related to human health that does not include human research subjects.
  - Clinical Research: Interventional and observational research designs that study human subjects in order to advance medical knowledge.
  - Medical Education Research: Clinical research design that investigates questions related to the understanding and improvement of medical education of healthcare professionals, patients, and others.
  - Global Health Research: Any of the above research designs that investigates issues related to global health or is done in an international setting.

10.3   When to Do Research: Start Early, Plan Ahead, Keep at It

Research is a skill that takes time and practice to develop. Thus, the best time to start research projects is now! The more experience a student has doing research, the more efficient and effective they will be. One challenge of the medical student researcher is balancing their medical school and extracurricular engagements with research projects. However, with the exception of possible dedicated research time during residency, this balancing act will continue for the rest of a student's career – balancing clinical, teaching, research, and administrative duties as well as obligations outside of the hospital such as family, friends, hobbies, and volunteerism. Thus, learning to time manage is another important aspect of engaging in research as a medical student. Below the years of medical school training are broken down to address specific time constraints, opportunities for research, and suggestions on prioritizing as a student tries to manage research with all other aspects of their training.

10.3.1   Pre-clinical Years: Time Manage, Prioritize

The first goal of any student beginning medical school should be to successfully transition to the rigor of medical school. Once a student feels accustomed to the pace and difficulty of their new curriculum, they should consider finding a research mentor and project. Often, medical schools will sponsor funded research time during the summer break between first and second year. However, students shouldn't let this dictate when they begin research projects. If they feel they can handle research in addition to their academic commitments, students should start seeking research projects in their first few months. See the above section on "Choosing a Research Area: Specialty" for more information on how to decide in what specialty a student should pursue their first research project.

First year of medical school offers many extracurricular opportunities. There is a wealth of student organizations and volunteer opportunities for first year medical students to get involved with. However, it is easy to become over-committed. Students should be judicious in what opportunities they pursue and how much time they commit to various organizations. A student should participate in a select number of organizations in order to develop leadership skills, serve their community, and/or pursue outside interests. The key is to have quality opportunities to learn and enjoy, while leaving adequate time for academics and, of course, research!

An integral part of the successful transition into medical training is learning to time manage and prioritize. Medical school learning is fast-paced, and commitments only increase as a one moves through training. Thus, learning to time-manage class obligations, extracurricular activities, and personal time with research projects is key. This skill will serve students well regardless of what field or area of work they decide to go into. Thus, while students should engage in research early in their medical school career, they should also start with smaller, manageable projects and work up to more time-intensive ones.

At the end of a student's pre-clinical years they take Step 1 of the United States Medical Licensing Exam. Scoring well on this exam is important for a successful residency application. Thus, students should heavily prioritize the 1–2 months leading up to this exam for adequate study. Those engaging in research should plan ahead and notify their mentors that they will have very limited time available for research projects during the time around Step 1. Research mentors who went to medical school or have worked with medical students in the past will undoubtedly understand the importance of this test and thus the time constraint, but students should make sure to notify mentors in advance.

It is important for student's to keep in mind that the pre-clinical years are often much more flexible than their clinical years. This schedule and freedom should be taken advantage of so that students are able to develop research and time management skills, in addition to the beginning of their research portfolio before entering the clinical years. Additionally, many medical schools offer summer breaks in between class during which students are encouraged to participate in career development activities. If available, students should absolutely capitalize on these times to focus on developing research projects and skills while they are not burdened by the demands of class or exams. There are often various funding opportunities from medical schools and professional organizations to support this work (see below section on "Funding Opportunities"). The possibility of an additional year in medical school, dedicated to research, will be discussed below (see below section on "Taking Additional Academic Time during Medical School"). Once students transition into the clinical years, they will not have as much time to complete projects so for many students the bulk of their research portfolio created in medical school is begun in their pre-clinical years.

10.3.2   *Clinical Years*

As with the transition into medical school, the transition into clinical years is an important time. Students should be prepared to substantially cut back on all commitments outside of their clinical duties, including research. Clinical years are a time when students are acquiring a vast amount of information daily on how to care for patients. It is essential that students set aside adequate time for independent study, clinical duties, and leisure time to remain balanced. Once a student feels they have become accustomed to the rigors of clinical training, they may decide to re-start smaller, less time-intensive research projects. Further, as their clinical training goes on, students will begin to have an understanding of which clinical rotations will be more or less demanding. Students can then plan ahead when they know they have a less time-intensive month to work on, start, or complete research projects during that time.

The clinical years also offer the opportunity for students to interact with faculty and residents of all different specialties in a one-on-one setting. If the opportunity is available, students should consider rotating on clerkships or services relevant to their research interests or with their research mentors. This allows the student to see the clinical side of the research they have been participating in as well as providing them with another setting in which to work with their research mentor.

Additionally, during clinical years students will have the opportunity to meet residents and faculty they were not exposed to in pre-clinical years. This is a great place to network in order to find new research mentorships and projects. For example, many surgical residents will complete dedicated research years mid-way through their training, so they are an excellent source of potential research and career mentors for students interested in academic surgery. Students should also take advantage of their interactions with residents to fully understand a specialty they may be interested in, including the research and training programs of the field.

The clinical years, by definition, also provide students with their first access to taking care of sick patients. At large academic hospitals, there are often unusual or rare cases. When appropriate, students may consider approaching residents or faculty regarding the possibility of assisting in writing a case report or literature review.

Many schools offer clinical students the opportunity to do research elective rotations during their clinical training. These are dedicated periods of time that students can engage in full-time research with a specified mentor. These months are particularly beneficial for students who have previously engaged in research projects, have established mentoring relationships, and have developed research skills that will allow them to be efficient in their work (all reasons to start early!). These research elective months can also be used for students to finalize projects or prepare others in their research group to take over should the student match for residency at another institution.

In the final year of medical school, students will be spend a large portion of time in the fall and/or winter traveling to interviews for residency. For residency interviews, students should be prepared to intelligently describe their various research projects – including the design, methods, and findings. A well-crafted research portfolio only benefits a student's application if they can truly demonstrate skills learned in creating it and an understanding of the work they have completed. Additionally, students who have spent several years completing various research projects may have an idea of their future research interests and goals. These goals will be helpful for students to evaluate programs that will best position them to have the type of academic career they are interested in. Students should evaluate the sort of support residents receive regarding research, the amount of residents participating in research, and the type of research being done at a given institution.

Summary
- Start early! Developing research skills and completing research projects takes time.
- Pre-clinical years are the ideal time to explore various research projects in order to gain skills and foster mentoring relationships with research faculty.
- Students should wisely considering priorities when agreeing to any commitments outside of their schoolwork and clinical duties, including research projects and extracurricular activities.
- Clinical years after more demanding than pre-clinical years, leaving less time for research.
- Take advantage of time that can be dedicated solely to research: summer after first year, clinical research electives.

10.4   Finding Research Mentors

10.4.1   What Makes a Good Mentee

The first step to finding a good research mentor, and thus creating a research portfolio, is for the student to first be a good mentee. The best mentees are those that are driven, enthusiastic, curious, honest, and self-reflective. They are students who are able to demonstrate to mentors a track record of success. There are some actionable steps students should take in order to be an efficient and effective mentee:

1. *Set clear goals*: Students should set clear goals for every encounter with anyone in the research team. These goals at times should be explicitly communicated to team members, while other times serve as personal benchmarks. Students should set goals for their research experience overall, and clearly communicate them to potential research mentors; for example, a student's goal may be to publish a first author paper. This will facilitate pairing of mentors and mentees whose goals and abilities are compatible. Students should continue to set smaller goals for every future encounter. At an update meeting, this may take the form of an agenda. At a lab meeting, this may take the form of personal learning objectives.

2. *Take initiative*: Time is a finite resource for everyone – research mentors especially. They often have clinical, teaching, and administrative duties in addition to serving as a research advisor for other professionals and staff. Mentees should take initiative to problem solve, answer their own questions, and complete work without extensive oversight. Students should seek out additional resources, when appropriate, before approaching their mentor. In this way students will learn to be self-starters, will progress through their projects more quickly, and will gain more skills.
3. *Don't be afraid to ask questions*: Part of taking initiative is taking the initiative to ask questions. Students should ask for help and ask to help: While it is important that students take initiative, they should also be honest and self-reflective regarding their own limitations. Students should ask for help when necessary. Beyond asking for assistance, students should ask members of the larger research team what they can do to be useful. When asking questions, students should keep two things in mind: (1) Have a clear objective – in other words, students should know specifically what they need when they approach a team member for help. (2) Come prepared – students should prepare to the extent to which they can so when they ask for help, they are clear and concise, and knowledgeable. For example, if a student needs help with a statistical analysis, they should know what the goal of this analysis is and specifically what question they are trying to answer. They should then read about various statistical methods in which to do this and to the best of their ability prepare their data so it is clean and ready to go.
4. *Be a team player*: Research, like surgery is a team sport. It is important that the student treat everyone with respect in the laboratory from administrative staff to undergraduate students, to technicians to more senior staff. Just like rotations, being in the laboratory is an audition for the next step of training.

10.4.2 *What Makes a Good Mentor*

In order to find a good mentor, a student must know what traits they are specifically seeking. The research mentor is one of the single most important components of a student's success in creating a research portfolio. First and foremost, a good research mentor is one who is interested and invested in the student and their goals. These are the mentors that will be available for students and committed to helping students get the resources they need to be successful in their research projects and career development. These mentors are often candid in their advice and feedback for students, and push them to grow as future researchers and clinicians. However, this quality is hard to intuit from a short, one-time meeting. Thus, students should employ specific strategies to best assess any future mentor:

1. Ask possible mentors about their history of mentoring previous students and/or residents. Faculty who enjoy mentoring trainees tend to do so regularly.

2. Ask possible mentors what resources they have to assist students in the research process – statisticians, staff research associates, research residents.
3. Ask possible mentors what their goals for the mentee would be to accomplish – such as presentations at conferences and publications. Students should also share what their goals would be.
4. Assess a possible mentor's productivity by looking for their number of publications. Specifically students should pay attention to the number of "in press" and recent publications, indicating an active group.
5. When looking at the possible mentor's recent publications, take note of the authorship. Who tends to be first author on the publications? Are there trainees in first, second, or third authorship positions?

Students should seek out research mentors who are productive and actively publishing with good resources available for student's development; such as full-time research associates, statisticians, and residents on research years. A full research team means there are more people with diverse backgrounds from which a student can learn and benefit. However, in order to be an effective mentor, a research mentor does not have to be publishing the most or have the biggest research group. The key is to find a mentor who is active, but also has the time to work with a medical student and provide mentorship. Of note, if a research mentor does not have staff statisticians available, many universities have statistical support available to faculty and students free of charge.

Just as students can seek research projects in other specialties as interests change, students should feel free to seek out other research mentorship opportunities should their needs change. However, it is important that students honor previous commitments and do not take on extra responsibilities on a new project unless they are able to also finish their previous ones. As stated above, the first step in finding a good research mentor and developing a research portfolio is for students to be good mentees.

10.4.3 How to Find That Research Mentor

There is no right or wrong way to find a research mentor. As mentioned above, by participating in research a student's network of potential research mentors may widen. Some may find their ideal research mentor at a national meeting, discussing a current project. Others may find a good research mentor while on a clinical rotation in their desired specialty. The below steps are simply to help students to get started especially in the first years in medical school.

#1. *Ask around*. The best resource a student has in finding a good research mentor is other students and faculty. Students should start by asking upperclassmen who have had successful research experiences in a specialty of interest for advice on what faculty to meet with and what projects might be good starting points. Another great resource is your surgery clerkship director. This member of the faculty has demonstrated a commitment to student success and will be knowledgeable about faculty in various departments who work well with students. While on your clinical rotations, residents are another great resource. By asking a variety of people, students will begin to create a list of potential mentors who will help them be successful.

#2. *Do your homework.* Once a student has a list of faculty that may be good potential research mentors, they should sit down and read up about their background and work. The student should assess the potential's productivity and the level to which students in their group contribute to publications, as mentioned above. Before contacting a potential mentor, students should have a good grasp of the mentor's research interests and recent publications.

#3. *Set up a meeting.* This is best done via a concise email that clearly establishes your goals and intentions. This will allow both the student and possible mentor to quickly evaluate whether there is a suitable match in terms of available projects, resources, and interests. See an example email below:

> Good afternoon Dr. Attending,
>
> I am a first year medical student looking to gain some research experience in the field of vascular surgery. Older Student, who worked with you during her second year on a project regarding outcomes following emergent aortic aneurysm repair, recommended I contact you given your history of excellent mentorship of successful medical students.
>
> I am looking for a research project and mentorship in clinical outcomes research in the field of vascular surgery. I would love to sit down and meet to discuss your research group, the project, and my goals. I have some experience in basic science research and have attached a recent CV for your review.
>
> Please let me know if you would be interested in meeting with me, and a time that is convenient for your schedule.
>
> Best regards,
> Eager Student

#4. *Prepare for the meeting.* Students should prepare for the meeting by first setting goals – what do they want to learn and accomplish. They should then review the potential mentor's research. Generally, academic medical centers will have websites with brief descriptions of a faculty's research interests. Start there for a broad overview. Next, read through the last few publications authored by a member of the mentor's group. Pay special attention to the knowledge gaps addressed by their work and to the methodology of their project. This will give students a good idea of how projects in this group are done and will prepare them to ask appropriate questions.

#5. *At the meeting.* Like any interview, students should be dressed professionally and prepared to take notes. At the meeting, students should be interested and engaged, and ready to talk about their current goals of a research project, their long-term goals, and their previous experiences. Keeping in mind they are new to this work, they should also express general enthusiasm for the research and a willingness to add value to the research group in ways the mentor sees fit. Short-term goals should be specific, but flexible, and relate to both learning objectives and productivity measures. Learning objectives might include learning particular study design, more about a disease topic, or practice with statistical analysis or writing. Even students with limited to no research experience should have some specific learning objective in mind. Productivity goals can include submission of abstracts for presentations at research conferences and authorship on manuscripts. Having specific objectives in mind will allow both mentor and mentee to quickly establish if this pairing would be beneficial for both parties.

Students should also be prepared to ask specific questions about the mentor (see section above, "What Makes a Good Mentor") and about potential projects. In the initial meeting, the mentor and/or mentee may not yet have a project in mind but it is important that as a project idea is developed the student asks questions and have a clear understanding of their role in the project. Specifics including expectations and timelines are important to clearly communicate. If you have no previous research experience, do not expect to be given a full project immediately as this would inappropriate and unfair to everyone.

When ending the meeting, the student should be gracious and conscientious of the mentor's time. The student should confirm the next steps and an appropriate timeline, so both mentor/mentee are on the same page about what comes next.

#6. *Follow up*. Following the meeting, a student should thank the potential mentor for taking time to meet with them – even if it was decided that they would not make a successful combination.

If the student is to work with the mentor, they should complete the next steps as discussed at the end of their meeting in a timely manner. Depending on the interaction, it may also be helpful to send a thank you email with a concise summary of the meeting to the research mentor; this can be beneficial in establishing the student's enthusiasm for working together, and can provide a useful summary for a busy faculty member.

The key of follow up, whatever it may be, is to be prompt. Delays of weeks between meetings and next step only detract valuable time that a student could be using to familiarize themselves with other research personnel, literature, or diving into a project. Delays may also signal to research mentors that the student does not have adequate time to dedicate to a given project or that the student is less committed than they are.

Summary

- The first step in finding a good mentor is to be a good mentee.
- Good mentees:

  - Are hard-working, enthusiastic, and honest.
  - Set clear goals.
  - Take initiative.
  - Ask questions.

- Good mentors have a history of mentoring, are committed to a student's success, and have ample opportunities for students to participate. Having a good mentor is critical to successfully building the research portfolio.
- To find a good mentor, start by asking peers and faculty who would be good potential mentors. Then employ the skills of a good mentee at every interaction.

10.5   Productivity in Research: The Research Portfolio

10.5.1   What Is "Productivity"?

Productivity in research, or "academic productivity," for medical students and residency applicants is largely regarded as the enumeration of abstracts, presentations, and publications and both the student's impact on the work (authorship) and the work's impact on the field. As one surgery chairman often tells his students, "They weigh them before they read them." A single paper in a very high impact journal such as the *New England Journal of Medicine* or *Nature* will be more impactful than several in the *Journal of Questionable Results*. Students should seek an experience that has the opportunity to publish in both high and low impact journals. Thus, productivity is a balance of quality in research and contribution and quantity. Over 70 % of students applying to general surgery residency in recent years have had at least one publication. Of those who were highly ranked by general surgery residencies, 93 % had some form of research experience (abstract, presentation, or publication) (Dort et al. 2015; Stain et al. 2013; Tchantchaleishvili et al. 2013). In integrated plastic surgery, applicants who matched had a mean of 12.5 abstracts, presentations, and publications (Borsting et al. 2015). In integrated cardiothoracic surgery, applicants had a median of 3 publications (Tchantchaleishvili et al. 2013).

Thus, students should seek to bring their research projects to submission of both abstracts for presentation and manuscripts. This is important because it disseminates the knowledge gained from the research project while adding to a student's research portfolio. Students should discuss with mentors to select the most appropriate academic conferences and journals to submit their work. To maximize both dissemination of knowledge and building of the research portfolio, students should make sure to submit work for both abstract presentation and manuscript publication. Additionally, medical students may be encouraged to submit their abstracts to multiple meetings (if the meeting so allows), to maximize the benefit of developing presentation skills, networking in large academic settings, and disseminate work.

Another measure of productivity is authorship of abstracts, presentations, and manuscripts. Students should seek to be highly involved in their research projects. First authorship indicates that the individual did the largest portion of the meaningful work related to a project. First authorship is an excellent goal for students engaged in research, especially after the successful completion of 1–2 smaller projects. However, any authorship is better than none, and students' research portfolios benefit greatly from any addition. Other ways to maximize a research portfolio is that a student, they may be able to be first author on an abstract presentation of part or all of the study at an academic meeting, even if they are not first author on the manuscript. This will give them the opportunity to develop their presentation skills as well as build meaningfully to their research portfolio.

10.5.2 How to Be Maximize Productivity: "Nights and Weekends Were Made for Reading and Writing"

Students can maximize productivity by ensuring that all research projects with which they are involved are submitted to relevant academic meetings (as determined by the research mentor) and submitted as a manuscript for publication. Students should work towards the goal of contributing meaningfully to all projects in which they are involved so as to gain important experience, contribute to the group, as well as achieve high-level authorship on research projects to augment their research portfolio. However, there are other, less direct actions that profoundly augment a student's research productivity: staying up-to-date with research in their field, investing time in developing key skills, setting realistic goals, and working smarter on research projects.

10.5.2.1 Staying Current with Literature

When first getting started in a new research area, students should ask their research mentor, other research staff, residents in the field, and other medical students for suggestions on papers to read to begin developing foundational knowledge. Excellent places to start include the research mentor's previous publications and major reviews published regarding your research field and topic. These will give you a nice introduction to the field, especially for pre-clinical students who may have limited exposure, as well as to the research design, methodology, and scientific questions of a given research mentor.

Once a student has developed baseline knowledge, the next step is to stay current with the research in their field; students should identify a few of the highest impact journals. This should be determined with the guidance of their research mentor, and are often the journals to which students should aspire to submit their work. Students should commit to reading every research abstract of articles published in these journals, and then reading the entire articles related to their specific areas of research – paying special attention to the methods and results sections. This will allow students to continue to build their understanding of the field and its direction, while introducing them to new advances, study design, and methodology relevant to their current (and future) projects.

Granted, all of the above reading is difficult to do on top of the many demands of medical school. Thus, at least in the beginning, students should take a structured approach. Students should set scheduled time aside each week to complete these readings. Once it becomes routine, students may find it is convenient to read an article in short bouts of empty space in their schedule: the 5 min break between lectures, on the bus ride home, while dinner is cooking. However, by having at minimum a set time aside each week, students will be able to stay current with the literature while establishing a routine that will likely serve them throughout their careers.

Staying current and knowledgeable about their field will contribute to a student's productivity and overall success in a number of ways. First of all, having a knowledge base for the field in which one is researching is essential to doing quality research. Beyond this, staying current and closely reading methods and results section of related research will help broaden a student's learning in their research experience beyond their own research project. Being up-to-date with the literature will make writing abstracts and manuscripts easier and more efficient; students will begin to get a sense of what high quality scientific writing looks like and will also be knowledgeable on what current publications would be relevant to cite in introduction and discussion sections of a manuscript. Lastly, in consistently reading the research breadth of the field, students will begin to develop their own ability to create and design relevant, impactful research questions – this means new projects and more productivity!

10.5.2.2 Investing in Essential Skills

In addition to dedicating time to gain background knowledge and stay current with the literature, students can improve their productivity by developing essential research skills early in their involvement. Developing these skills will serve students in their research careers in medical school and beyond. This means students should get involved with every step in the research process that they can: grant writing, study design, laboratory work, statistical analysis, presentations, poster creation, and manuscript writing. The more students do in these areas, the easier it will be able to complete them for later projects. While it may be easier or seem faster to ignore the steps that another research team member completed, by investing time in understanding the full process students will develop skills that will make them more self-sufficient and more efficient in future research projects.

For example, many research groups may have staff statisticians to help with data analysis. Students will gain much more if they ask to sit down with the statistician to discuss the analysis and ask questions rather than just taking the results and plugging them into a paper. By understanding the process, the student will be better equipped to present the study whether that's on a poster, in an oral presentation, or as a manuscript. Thus, saving time in the back-and-forth later down the line. Plus, this opportunity will allow the student to learn more skills in statistical analysis than they would have otherwise.

10.5.2.3 Goal Setting

This chapter has touched upon goal setting in various regards, including as students prepare to seek out research projects, as they meet with mentors, and as they begin to work on projects. In this last area, goal setting can be extraordinarily useful in increasing a student's productivity. Students should have larger goals in mind with a given project, but they should set shorter-term goals to work towards their larger aspirations. The timing of this can be individualized based on a given student's needs, but setting weekly or monthly goals is a good place to start. Additionally, having goals set to be achieved by the next mentor-mentee meeting is another added layer of accountability for students and mentors to ensure that work is progressing and appropriate steps are being taken.

There is an abundance of literature and research on goal setting that student's can explore. In this section, we will briefly detail one commonly used method to approach goal setting: SMART criteria. SMART stands for: Specific, Measureable, Achievable, Relevant, Time-bound (Doran 1981).

- **Specific**: Set specific, rather than general, goals. Specific goals can answer the following 5 questions:

  - What do I want to accomplish?
  - Why is this a worthy goal?
  - Who will be involved?
  - Where will this take place?
  - How will I be able to accomplish this?

- **Measureable**: Goals need to have a concrete way to measure progress and success. This will allow students to stay on track or to ask for help if they are unable to stay on track. A measurable goal will be able to answer: How will I know when I am halfway to my goal?
- **Achievable**: Desired goals should be realistic and attainable. Students should be clear with mentors about their goals and get feedback on whether their goals are achievable given their individual constraints of skills, resources, time, etc.
- **Relevant**: The basis of the relevant tenet is the question: Does this goal matter? In other words, in setting goals, students should make sure that what they are working towards is worthy of the time and effort being put in.
- **Time-bound**: Lastly, a goal that is measurable and achievable should be put on a time-frame. This will allow deliberate self-reflection and accountability regarding these goals. A time-bound goal can answer the question: When am I halfway to my goal?

As students set goals for their research, they should do so in conjunction with goals for other aspects of their life and schooling. This will allow the goals to be realistic with the individual commitments or needs a student may have. In working with mentors to set goals and be held accountable for them, students and mentors will also be able be realistic with the student's current abilities and needs in order to be successful at achieving the larger goals at hand of finishing the project, learning something new, and publishing their work.

Thus, by setting SMART short-term goals that work towards a longer-term goal, students are kept on track and able to measure their progress. This will increase their ability to be productive even during their busiest times in medical school.

10.5.2.4   Working Smarter Towards Publication

Begin with the end in mind. The final goal of any research project is a manuscript for publication. Thus, when a student is designing a research question with a mentor, they should try to envision how they would want the manuscript regarding that question to read.

- What is already known and published regarding this topic?
- What is not known about this topic?
- What main study question would this project address?
- What other questions would be interesting?
- What figures might be useful to illustrate these type of results?

In this way, the mentor/mentee pair can anticipate the types of experiments or analyses that need to be completed for a thorough manuscript that addresses their original question.

In preparing for a research project, a student will undoubtedly conduct a thorough review of the current literature on the topic. It is essential before starting a project for the student to understand what has been answered in relation to this question already. While completing this review, a student should begin to craft an annotated bibliography in a systematic way. Each individual may have their preferences, but there are key elements from every paper that students should include in this bibliography:

- Publication Information

    - Title
    - First Author, Principal Author
    - Journal
    - Publication year

- Study Design

    - Research question
    - Overview of methods, relevant to the scientific discipline of the study

- Main Results

By doing this in a systematic, organized way for every relevant paper a student reads, they will end up with not only an in-depth understanding of the literature available on the topic, but will have a useful reference for writing their manuscript or quickly reviewing the literature when giving a presentation later.

The other key towards working smarter towards a publication is starting writing early. Many students new to research come in with the belief that manuscript preparation begins once the experiment and analysis is complete. However, the most efficient, productive researchers are writing at every step in the process.

Once the literature review has been completed and the main question of the research project defined, the student should work on writing the introduction of the manuscript. Before they lift a pipette or run their first T-test, they should have a cursory introduction written. The reason for this is that the student will be the most familiar with the literature at this point, which makes the task of writing the introduction much easier. It will also force the student to ensure that their research question is clearly defined and they understand the project well.

The next step is to write a brief outline of the methods section. This section will evolve as the research project occurs, but writing out the methods a student plans to use before ever starting the project will help to ensure that the research design is sound and complete; this may catch and/or prevent errors of methodology, which could lead to having to repeat parts of the project. As the student (finally) begins the actual research process, they should be referencing this methods section of their future manuscript frequently – revising and adding as appropriate. This way no step of the experiment or analysis is lost. Ultimately, when revising the final manuscript, the student can then make the methods section clear and concise, using the draft they created throughout the project.

Thus, by the time a student finishes a research project and prepares to sit down and write up their results in a manuscript, they already have drafts of two of the four sections done! This will allow students to be efficient in their research processes, which translates into producing more publishable work, and building up their research portfolios.

Summary

- Productivity is often measured by the quantity and quality of a student's abstracts, presentations, and manuscripts
- Students can maximize productivity by

  - Staying current with literature in their field
  - Investing in essential research skills
  - Setting SMART short-term and long-term goals
  - Working smarter towards a manuscript

10.6 Funding Opportunities

Applying for funding for a research project is an important way that students can gain important skills about literature review and grant writing, while building up their research portfolio. Research grants and awards, in addition to publications and presentations, are great ways for students to enhance their research portfolio and residency applications. Thus, at every opportunity, students should seek funding opportunities for research projects; specifically, students should seek funding opportunities for dedicated research time such as a summer vacation.

Most medical schools keep up-to-date lists of funding opportunities that apply to and/or are geared specifically towards medical students. Medical schools themselves often provide funding for their students to pursue research during summer vacations. These are excellent sources of funding if others cannot be attained.

Students should sit down with their mentors and medical school representatives to discuss any funding awards that might suit their projects. Students can begin their searches by looking at specialty societies, the American Medical Association, the National Institutes of Health, state health organizations, and private not-for-profit agencies.

Summary
- Funding opportunities enhance a student's research portfolio
- Students should seek funding opportunities at every opportunity

10.7   Taking an Additional Academic Time During Medical School

Many students with a passion for research grapple with the question of taking additional time during medical school to complete dedicated research time. This may take the form of additional degrees or time dedicated solely to research. Additional degrees can provide students with additional skills and knowledge to pursue more complex research questions. There are benefits and disadvantages to each path. This is a highly individual decision that a student should make after carefully considering their career goals and discussing the prospects in depth with trusted mentors and advisers.

Some possibilities are outlined in the table below. Please note, this list is not extensive and other programs such as Masters in Health Science or Masters in Clinical Research exist. Students should consider how their long-term career goals align with the various options, including the decision to not take time for additional training during their medical school career. Various funding routes should also be taken into consideration – for example, most MD/PhD students will have funding for their PhD and remaining years of medical school, while MPH and MBA funding may be harder to secure. When making this decision, students should also keep in mind the possibility to pursue these degrees during and after residency. Lastly, when applying to highly competitive surgical fields, students and mentors may feel that by having an additional year to complete research or pursue a degree of interest may help them be successful in the residency application process. All of these individual circumstances and more should be considered and discussed with a knowledgeable mentor, as well as family members, medical school advisors, and/or deans.

Summary
- The decision of whether to take additional academic time to pursue another degree or a dedicated research year is extremely individual
- Students should evaluate their career and research goals and meet with experienced mentors and educators regarding their decision
- Options include, but are not limited to, PhD, MPH, MBA, or dedicated research year without additional degrees.

	Description	Benefits	Disadvantages	Who should consider
Doctors of Philosophy (PhD)	A PhD is awarded to students after completion of coursework in their field and a dissertation based on extensive original research.	Unparalleled academic training in a specific research field. PhD students will have dedicated research years with training under guidance of a seasoned research faculty.	This pathway is the most time-intensive. Most students add an additional 4 years to their training. You must decide early on topics, which often results in research in a different area than final specialty.	A student with a deep interest in an academic career heavily focused on research.
Masters in Public Health (MPH)	An MPH is a multidisciplinary professional degree that includes areas of study relevant to public health, such as biostatistics, epidemiology, social science, environmental health, policy, and behavioral science.	MPH is excellent training for students with particular interests in public health research and epidemiology.	This multidisciplinary degree is earned in 1 year while covering a wide array of subjects, so a student may not get in depth training in a specific interest nor have much time to complete hands-on research.	A student committed to working and conducting research in areas of public health
Masters in Business Administration (MBA)	An MBA is a degree aimed to develop skills required for management, leadership, and business. Students will study accounting/economics, management, marketing, and operations along with elective courses where students can pursue individual interests.	MBA training offers medical students a unique set of skills to approach medicine from a business perspective. For students with particular interest in business, management, and systems research, this degree may be ideal.	An MBA is not aimed to prepare students for a career in research, and thus serves a specific interest area. Additionally, the degree time itself is often very time-consuming, preventing students from having much dedicated research time.	A student interest in business, hospital administration, and systems research.
Research year	A dedicated year of full time research that a student pursues as part of a pre-existing yearlong fellowship or in conjunction with a mentor and research group.	Aside from pursuing a PhD, this option allows students the most time to focus on completing research projects. Allows development of a new skill that will set them apart from peers.	There may not be any formalized training, so students will need to seek out opportune mentors who can provide guidance as well as seek out individual learning opportunities.	A student with a particular research interest, a strong research mentor, and a desire to enter residency with a foundational research skills.

10.8 Packaging the Research Portfolio

After years of hard work and dedication, medical students will prepare their applications to residency. By this time, students will hopefully have created a research portfolio of which they can be proud. They have hopefully learned a great deal about their research area, the scientific method, study design, laboratory and statistical techniques, and writing/presenting scientific work. Their research throughout medical school will likely have prepared them to be productive in their residencies, fellowships, and beyond. Research is an essential component to application to surgical residency. Over 70 % of students to general surgery applying will have at least one publication; and this number only increases for competitive sub-specialties. The only question left is – how can these skills be best expressed during the residency application process?

There are four areas in which research abilities and accomplishments can be highlighted:

1. Personal statement
2. Letters of recommendation
3. Curriculum vita
4. Interviews

The first opportunity is the student's personal statement. This is a page-long document that addresses why a student is interested in the field, what they are looking for in a residency program, and what the student's goals are in their chosen field long-term (Gonzalez 2016). Beyond these three aims, a personal statement should highlight what strengths a student would bring to the program in concrete ways. Thus, a student should think about each of these goals of the personal statement and carefully consider the ways in which their research may apply. For example, their research experience may have been integral to a student's decision to pursue that specialty, may be a significant component by which a student will evaluate programs, and/or may drive their long-term career goals. However, regardless of the aim research addresses, a student should always use the opportunity to highlight the knowledge, experience, and skills they have developed through research and why that would make them an excellent residency candidate. This should be done through concrete, concise examples. By addressing their research experience in the personal statement in clear but succinct ways, the student will help tie together their curriculum vitae and will create the opportunity to describe these research experiences during interviews.

The next area for consideration is a student's letters of recommendation (LOR). Students applying to general surgery have four LOR total, one of which must come from the department chair. Thus, three LOR are selected by the student. The student should seek out letter writers who can comment on a student's clinical abilities, professionalism, and research experience. A letter writer should be someone willing to provide strong support. With select exceptions, letter writers for students applying to surgical disciplines should be clinicians with experience in the field that the student is applying. Thus, students should consider whether their research mentors fit the above criteria. Research mentors with whom students have worked with clinically and are leaders in their field are optimal letter writers because their letters will be respected by their colleagues, and they will be able to comment personally on both clinical and research abilities of the student. However, many research mentors may not be ideal letter writers; they may not be clinicians, may be in a different specialty, or may not have worked with a student clinically. For letter writers not familiar with a student's research background, a student should provide a complete curriculum vita (CV) and emphasize their research experience, skills, and accomplishments when meeting with letter writers. In meetings with potential letter writers, students should emphasize their research experience and highlight the skills they have gained and their subsequent research accomplishments.

A student's CV may include the following areas related to their research: Research Publications, Research Presentations, Research Experience, Honors and Awards, Professional Memberships. The key here is for students to list all relevant and applicable items on their CV. Students should be very careful to accurately cite their experiences and not modify or exaggerate. This is a well-known phenomenon and residency programs are apt to look for this. This includes falsifying publications, altering authorship, etc. Students should approach their CV with integrity and honesty, while maximizing the experiences they listed.

- *Research Publications*: Students should list all publications in peer-reviewed journals of which they have been an author, in chronological order. This includes all journals indexed on PubMed as well as special interest journals such as medical student research journals.
- *Research Presentations*: Students should list all presentations of which they have had authorship. These presentations can be at regional, national, or international meetings of established organizations and departments. This includes both poster and oral presentations. Students should list oral presentations and posters for which they were not the presenter, but were an author.
- *Research Experience*: This is the place where students can describe all research experiences they have had – both those that led to publications/presentations and those that did not. In this area students should be prepared to describe the duration, their mentors, their responsibilities, and their accomplishments during the research experience.
- *Honors and Awards*: This section can also emphasize a student's research accomplishments. Any grants that students were awarded to support their research or research growth (e.g. travel grants for meetings) should be included. Students should also include any awards won for their research, whether it be for a specific project or for a research portfolio overall.
- *Professional Memberships*: It is likely that after engaging in the research community, students will be members of professional societies at which they have presented, applied for grants, or attended meetings. These can also be highlighted on a student's CV.

Lastly, students with quality applications will be invited to interview at residency programs. Residency interviews are very important in the application process and students should approach them with substantial preparation. From a research portfolio perspective, students should review all items listed on their CV and be prepared to talk about each in detail. Students should be able to discuss their contribution to the work, the question addressed by the study, the methods used, and the results and implications. Again, students should not misrepresent the extent of their involvement in a project; however, students should be knowledgeable about the project overall regardless of their level of involvement. Further, students should see questions about their research as opportunities to highlight the skills they have developed through these works. Thus, a question about a summer research project turns into the opportunity for the student to discuss how their ability to write a manuscript evolved or how they learned to work in a multidisciplinary team. Finally, students will get a variety of broad interview questions for which concrete research examples may be useful. Questions regarding a candidate's challenges, failures, accomplishments are all well suited to highlight research experiences and skills developed.

Summary

- Students should present their research portfolio in residency applications with integrity and honesty
- Personal Statement: Students should maximize their residency applications by using concrete examples of research experience in their personal statements
- Letters of Recommendation:

  - Students should consider asking for LOR from research mentors who are clinicians and can comment on their clinical abilities
  - Students should highlight research experience to letter writers who are unfamiliar

- Curriculum Vita:

  - Students should include publications, presentations, research experience, awards, and professional memberships, as applicable
  - Students should never alter author order or falsify publications/presentations on their CV

- Interviews:

  - Students should be prepared to discuss any research listed on their CV or personal statement in interviews
  - Students should use questions about specific research projects as an opportunity to highlight skills developed or accomplishments
  - Students should consider using concrete research examples as answers to generic interview questions

10.9   Conclusion

Participating in research is an excellent way for medical students to contribute to their profession, develop essential academic and non-academic skills, and become desired candidates for residency application. There are many types of research in which students can engage from basic to clinical research, in various specialties, and in various settings. Students interested in surgery, research, and/or developing important skills should seek out research opportunities early in their medical careers and continue to incorporate research throughout their education. Students should first look to themselves to be honest, enthusiastic, driven mentees and then look for invested research mentors who have the time and resources to help develop a student. Students can make the most of their research experiences by staying current with research in their field and participating in all aspects of the project. By setting realistic and measurable goals, students can become productive researchers and complete many presentations and publications. Students can also develop their research portfolio by applying for funding for their research projects. Students particularly interested in developing specific skills and having more thorough research experiences may consider taking time away from medical school to pursue additional degrees or full-time research. Ultimately, students should use their research portfolio to their advantage when applying for residency, making sure to highlight and emphasize their experiences, accomplishments, and skills in all aspects of the application process.

References

Borsting EA, Chim JH, Thaller SR. An updated view of the integrated plastic surgery match. Ann Plast Surg. 2015;75(5):556–9.

Doran GT. There's a S.M.A.R.T. way to write management's goals and objectives. Manag Rev (AMA FORUM). 1981;70(11):35–6.

Dort JM, Trickey AW, Kallies KJ, Joshi AR, Sidwell RA, Jarman BT. Applicant characteristics associated with selection for ranking at independent surgery residency programs. J Surg Educ. 2015;72(6):e123–9.

Gonzalez J. Writing your personal statement. Transitioning to Residency 2016. 2016. http://www. ama-assn.org/ama/pub/about-ama/our-people/member-groups-sections/minority-affairs-section/transitioning-residency/writing-your-personal-statement.page?. Accessed 1 Jan 2016.

Stain SC, Hiatt JR, Ata A, et al. Characteristics of highly ranked applicants to general surgery residency programs. JAMA Surg. 2013;148(5):413–7.

Stringer MD, Ahmadi O. Famous discoveries by medical students. ANZ J Surg. 2009;79(12):901–8.

Tchantchaleishvili V, Barrus B, Knight PA, Jones CE, Watson TJ, Hicks GL. Six-year integrated cardiothoracic surgery residency applicants: characteristics, expectations, and concerns. J Thorac Cardiovasc Surg. 2013;146(4):753–8.

The General Surgery Milestone Project. Accreditation Council for Graduate Medical Education and American Board of Surgery, 2015 July; 2015.

Chapter 11
Exposure to Academic Surgery as a Medical Student

Jacob A. Greenberg

Abstract Medical students are exposed to a diverse array of specialties and sub-specialties during their third year clerkship. Within surgery, they may be exposed to a variety of practice settings as well including private and community practice or academic surgery. For those interested in pursuing a career in academic surgery it is often beneficial to maximize your exposure to surgery during your time in medical school. This chapter will review several opportunities to increase your exposure to academic surgery as a medical student.

11.1 Introduction

It has been shown that early exposure to surgery and to members of the surgical faculty significantly increases interest in pursuing a surgical career, but for many students, gaining exposure to surgery early in medical school seems like a daunting task. While it may not be possible to go to the operating room on the first day of medical school, there are a variety of opportunities for medical students to gain exposure to academic surgery prior to their surgical clerkship rotation. This chapter will review many of the opportunities to experience academic surgery as a medical student, including funding opportunities for research, involvement in surgical societies, and identifying a mentor in academic surgery.

11.2 Institutional Opportunities

For students looking for exposure to surgery, the first place to start is at one's own institution. While opportunities for pre-clinical surgical exposure are institutional dependent, there are several that are available to students at most medical schools.

J.A. Greenberg (✉)
University of Wisconsin, Madison, WI, USA
e-mail: greenbergj@surgery.wisc.edu

© Springer International Publishing Switzerland 2017
M.J. Englesbe, M.O. Meyers (eds.), *A How To Guide For Medical Students*,
Success in Academic Surgery, DOI 10.1007/978-3-319-42897-0_11

11.2.1 Educational Conferences

All departments of surgery at academic institutions have some form of educational conference on a regular basis. The Morbidity and Mortality Conference is an educational and quality improvement conference that provides the surgical faculty with an opportunity to discuss operations that led to a complication. These difficult cases are discussed in detail to determine what could be done differently in order to prevent similar complications in the future. Attendance at this conference provides insight into how academic surgeons think about quality of care and improving their own performance and decision-making in the care of their patients.

Grand Rounds is another educational opportunity that is open to attendance by medical students. During Grand Rounds, a variety of local and national surgeons and researchers will present a topic of their choice that is pertinent to the field of surgery. The clinical topics will likely be of greatest interest to medical students and provide an opportunity to hear about research that is being conducted by surgeons at that institution. This could lead to the opportunity to work with that particular surgeon on a research project as a medical student.

In addition to these larger educational offerings, many surgical subspecialties will have either individual or multi-disciplinary conferences that focus on a specific set of diseases. For example, there may be a hepatobiliary conference that includes surgical oncologists, medical oncologists, radiation oncologists, and radiologists to review the treatment plans of patients with malignant diseases of the liver and pancreas. These conferences are an excellent educational opportunity for students with distinct surgical interests. They are often smaller than Morbidity and Mortality or Grand Rounds and provide students with the opportunity to form meaningful relationships with members of the surgical faculty.

11.2.2 Surgical Interest Groups

Most medical schools have some form of a student run surgical interest group. These groups serve to expose first and second year students to the practice of surgery as well as to members of the surgical faculty. Most groups meet once a month to discuss topics that are pertinent to medical students. Often, these sessions focus on a surgeon's own practice so they can discuss what life is like as a trauma or transplant surgeon. Others sessions will focus on suturing and knot tying or mock interviews for residency programs. The yearly agenda is created by the students and is molded to fit the needs of the group. There are often social events to provide students with the opportunity to meet and get to know members of the surgical faculty outside of the hospital. Participation and leadership of these groups can be both rewarding as well as an excellent opportunity to find a surgical mentor.

11.2.3 Shadowing Opportunities

Policies regarding students shadowing surgical faculty members in clinics and the operating room are variable. Surgery interest groups may be able to provide students with information regarding this opportunity. Students are also encouraged to reach out to a faculty member of interest and see if they would be willing to have first and second year students accompany them during a clinical experience. Students who have the opportunity to shadow a faculty member should present themselves in a professional manner by arriving promptly and appropriately attired. These experiences can be formative and provide students with an opportunity to form a longer and deeper relationship with a member of their surgical faculty.

11.2.4 Senior Medical Student Programs

For the majority of students, the real introduction to academic surgery comes during the third and fourth year surgical rotations and participation in a surgical bootcamp. These topics will be covered in greater detail in Chaps. 7 and 8, respectively. Several academic institutions across the country offer dedicated programs to senior medical students interested in pursuing a surgical career. The University of Michigan offers an annual "Student Surgery Leadership Weekend" in the spring (http://surgeryleadershipweekend.umich.edu). This program focuses on creating future leaders in academic surgery. Sessions include leadership workshops, mock residency interviews, and tips for matching in a surgical residency.

11.3 Surgical Societies

There are a tremendous number of surgical societies and navigating them as a medical student can be a daunting task. While most of these societies have some form of membership for students and residents, many are focused on providing updates in clinical care to surgeons in practice and may not have significant educational opportunities focused on medical students. While all of them will provide at least some exposure to academic surgery, there are a handful of societies that have medical student programs.

11.3.1 The American College of Surgeons

The American College of Surgeons (ACS) is the largest surgical society in the United States. Medical students may become members of the ACS by completing an online application (https://www.facs.org/member-services/join/medical-student)

and submitting a $20 application fee. Beyond this application fee, there are no annual dues for medical students. The Clinical Congress, the annual meeting of the ACS, is held annually in October. This meeting is an opportunity to hear updates in clinical practice, scientific research, surgical education, and a variety of other topics.

In addition to the scientific program at the Clinical Congress, there is a three-day program dedicated to medical students. This program is open to students in all 4 years of medical school and is designed for students interested in pursuing a career in surgery. The program includes a variety of topics including lifestyle issues in surgery and strategies for applying to surgical residencies. There is a medical student poster session where 40 students are able to share their surgical research with their peers. The program provides students with an opportunity to network with other medical students interested in surgery, surgical residents from a variety of programs across the country, general surgery residency Program Directors and Departmental Chairs, as well as leaders of the ACS. The program concludes with a cocktail reception for students and residency Program Directors. Medical Student members of the ACS may attend this program free of charge with advanced registration, while student non-members must pay an enrollment fee.

11.3.2 Association for Academic Surgery

The Association for Academic Surgery (AAS) is the largest academic surgical society in the United States and is focused on inspiring and developing young academic surgeons. It is an innovative and energetic society that has much to offer medical students with an interest in surgery. One of the major focuses of the AAS is mentorship, and medical students can easily find academic surgical mentors from a variety of different specialties and research interests. Medical student membership in the AAS requires an annual dues payment of $15 with the option of paying an additional $50 for a subscription to the *Journal of Surgical Research*.

The Academic Surgical Congress is an annual meeting of both the AAS and the Society of University Surgeons (SUS), another major academic surgical society. It is held in early February and has a diverse program with separate tracks focusing on Basic and Translational Research, Health Services and Outcomes Research, and Education Research. The Academic Surgical Congress is an outstanding opportunity for medical students to present their work, as there are a combination of poster sessions, full oral podium presentations, and briefer Quickshot oral presentations. There are opportunities to meet the leadership of the AAS and SUS as well as a Mentor/Mentee breakfast where medical students are paired with mentors from the two represented societies.

11.3.3   Association for Surgical Education

The Association for Surgical Education (ASE) is a national organization focused on researching and improving the state of surgical education in the United States and worldwide. While the organization has interest in the entire spectrum of surgical education, there is a strong focus on medical student and resident education. Membership for medical students costs $50 annually.

The ASE meets annually during "Surgical Education Week" which is a joint meeting along with the Association for Program Directors in Surgery. Sessions at the meeting are focused on the science and implementation of innovative educational programs in surgical training. As with others societies, there are ample networking opportunities in order to facilitate identification of a potential mentor in academic surgery. The ASE offers several Surgery Education Research Fellowship (SERF) positions annually. The SERF program is a 1-year fellowship where fellows are assigned a mentor through the ASE to assist in the creation and completion of a research project in surgical education. Recipients of the fellowship are expected to present their work during Surgical Education Week and are encouraged to publish their work in a surgical journal.

11.4   Research Funding

The primary focus of medical students should be to learn the tremendous volume of information required to complete medical school and prepare for residency training. However, many medical schools provide students with opportunities to perform research concurrently with their studies or over the summer between their first and second year. While research opportunities and requirements vary between institutions, it is worthwhile for students to know what resources may be available to support their research endeavors.

11.4.1   Institutional Resources

Many departments of surgery have grant support through their institution for summer research programs to be completed between the first and second year of medical school. For example, at the University of Wisconsin, the Shapiro Summer Research Fellowship allows nearly half of the medical students to perform research with a faculty member in one of the many departments throughout the medical school. In the department of surgery, students identify mentors from a list of projects and spend the summer months working with their faculty mentor on a research project that often culminates with a presentation at a national meeting and authorship on a manuscript. This type of interaction exposes students to the basics of medical research in basic and translation sciences, health services, education, or clinical outcomes, and also exposes them to members of the surgical faculty at their local institution.

11.4.2 National Resources

There are also a variety of federal and societal funding sources for medical students to support both short periods of research as well periods of up to 1-year of dedicated research time. The National Institutes of Health T35 grant is a short-term research grant that provides support for students in health professional schools to perform research over the summer or during off quarters. Several medical societies such as the American Medical Association and the Alpha Omega Alpha Honor Medical Society also have annual applications for research grants that are open to medical students.

11.5 Identifying a Mentor in Surgery

Identifying a positive role model as a mentor can be beneficial for a variety of personal and professional reasons. Mentors provide students with exposure to all aspects of academic surgery, help them through the residency application process, and even continue to mentor them through their residency and professional career. While most academic surgeons recognize the importance of mentorship and are honored to serve as a mentor to medical students and residents, they will generally not seek out a mentee. Medical students must be proactive and seek out their own mentor.

For most medical students, their surgical mentor will be a faculty member that they develop a close relationship with during their 3rd year clerkship in surgery or their 4th year surgical sub-internship. While identifying a mentor earlier in medical school is possible, it is often difficult to form a meaningful relationship with a faculty member outside of research projects during the pre-clinical years (Identifying a research mentor will be covered in greater detail in Chap. 9: Developing a Research Portfolio as a Medical Student). Medical students are encouraged to maximize their time with this faculty member and work with them in all possible clinical and didactic settings. Students should also arrange for regular meetings with their faculty mentor to discuss their own professional goals and to plan for their application to general surgery residency programs. Surgical residents can also serve as excellent mentors to medical students. Students and residents will work closely together during the 3rd and 4th year and students will have the opportunity to observe what life as a surgical resident is like.

While this may seem like a daunting task to many students, most faculty members and residents view the mentoring of students as part and parcel of their professional duties. Students should seek out mentorship early and continue to develop the relationship with their mentor whenever possible.

11.6 Summary

Gaining exposure to academic surgery early in medical school can have a profound impact on a student's professional goals. There are a wide variety of institutional and national opportunities for students to be involved in academic surgery. The more proactive students are in seeking out these opportunities, the more likely they will be to benefit from them.

Suggested Readings

AAS for Medical Students and Residents: http://www.aasurg.org/aasforstudents.php

American College of Surgeons. The value of membership for the medical student. https://www.facs.org/~/media/files/member%20services/member%20benefits/medicalstudentbenefits.ashx

Healy NA, Cantillon P, Malone C, Kerin MJ. Role models and mentors in surgery. Am J Surg. 2012;204:256–61.

Part III
The Residency Search and Match

Chapter 12
Preparing to Apply and Choosing a Specialty

Karole T. Collier and Rachel R. Kelz

Abstract This chapter will provide key information on the match process and outline basic information on surgical specialties. The following sections include tips for the successful assessment of one's competitiveness as a surgical residency candidate, and offer a guide to a successful surgical residency match for applicants early in their medical career.

12.1 Introduction

Surgeons often define themselves by the type of surgery that they perform. Each specialty has its own personality. The scope of practice will often define the type of patients treated, research interests, societies of membership, and the bulk of one's professional activities. For that reason, choosing a residency program remains inextricably linked to your personal passions and daily motivations. You need to pick a specialty that suits your personality and style. Find a place where you belong and you feel at home.

To become successful in the surgical residency match, you must be able to say more than just, "I want to be a surgeon". You will need to explain your motivations beyond simply becoming a surgeon. You need to be able to articulate, "why surgery?" Your answer should include information on the specific surgical field of your choice or plans to help you identify a specialty during residency. You should focus on your journey to surgery and reveal specific moments in time that led to your decision to become a surgeon. Your story should include more than just clinical facts. Build from your entire history, weave the facts together, and permit people to appreciate the appropriateness of your decision to pursue surgical training.

The match process can be intimidating. Hopefully, you have managed yourself well during medical school, and as such, your candidacy for the right program will be excellent. However, not everyone has a perfect record. In fact, most students do not, so don't freak out if you are in the middle of the pack. Enter the match with

K.T. Collier • R.R. Kelz (✉)
University of Pennsylvania, Philadelphia, PA, USA
e-mail: Karole.Collier@uphs.upenn.edu; Rachel.Kelz@uphs.upenn.edu

© Springer International Publishing Switzerland 2017
M.J. Englesbe, M.O. Meyers (eds.), *A How To Guide For Medical Students,*
Success in Academic Surgery, DOI 10.1007/978-3-319-42897-0_12

realistic expectations. Listen carefully when you meet with your advisors, and take note of what they tell you about your competitiveness. Factor this information into the types and number of programs to which you apply.

While many points of data go into evaluation of a student applying to surgery residency program, common metrics include United States Medical Licensing Exam (USMLE) Step 1 and 2 scores, 3rd year clerkship grades (particularly surgery), Alpha Omega Alpha (AOA) status and strength of letters of recommendation. Many programs additionally take into account whether a student has been involved in research. Being involved early in your medical school career with mentors in surgery can help you develop both research productivity, and relationships with people who can provide you with a strong letter of recommendation. For many medical students, an easy way to evaluate the competitiveness of their application is to assess their record and accomplishments. One way to organize this is listed in Table 12.1. The acronym P.A.P.E.R.S is a useful tool in organizing your strengths and weaknesses. Think honestly about your past performance overall (P), academic record (A), passion(s) for work (P), extracurricular activities (E), research accomplishments (R) and special circumstances (S). The PAPERS acronym addresses some of the concrete attributes that programs seek in a stellar applicant. It will help you catalogue your career to this point and journal it in the Electronic Residency Application System (ERAS) for review by the residency programs.

You will need to set aside some dedicated time in your 2nd and/or 3rd year of medical school to manage the application process. This means planning your elective schedule so that you can get letters of recommendations from people in your chosen field. This is also time to make sure you are happy with your choice of specialties. You should be organized and ask for letters early in the process as your mentors and faculty are busy and they will not be able to make deadlines if you do not give them advanced warning. All the while work on your application. Gather the information required, write your personal statement and start to investigate programs online. If you choose surgery late in the game, it just means that you will have to accelerate the pace of these activities.

12.2 Surgical Specialties

The surgical specialty that you choose may influence your candidacy. Some specialties are more competitive than others in part just because of supply and demand in the field and the number of residency spots. Any of these specialties can lead to a career in academic surgery and may combine aspects of surgical practice, research and teaching. For the student who is reading this early in their medical career, a brief review of the major fields of general surgery, as well as surgical specialties, is provided for your information.

Table 12.1 The Acronym PAPERS designed to catalogue your accolades

Past performance overall (P)	Childhood background
	Complete college record
	Nontraditional activities prior to medical school
	Awards, scholarships, travel
	Post-baccalaureate performance
Academic record (A)	Medical school grades/rank[a]
	USMLE Step 1 Score[a]
	USMLE Step 2 Score
	Step 2 CK performance
	AOA
	Honor societies
	Awards
Passion(s) for work (P)	What drives you?
	What have you accomplished in the domain that you love best?
	What tangible proof do you have that you can perform well when you are really motivated?
Extracurricular activities (E)	Include everything that you will be willing to discuss in an interview (clubs, community service, sports, culinary activities, work outside of medical student responsibilities, travel including global health experiences etc.)
	Summarize each activity succinctly without losing the ability to communicate its meaning
	Make sure your summary communicates what you have done to someone who is not familiar with the activities
	Highlight leadership positions
Research accomplishments (R)	Include duration of your commitment to each setting
	Abstracts, papers, presentations
	Awards, honors, grants
	Authorship position
	Role in projects (make sure this is confirmed or supported by a letter of recommendation by your PI)
Special circumstances (S)	Exceptional accomplishments
	Blemishes to your record
	Specific challenges that affected your performance
	Any gaps that you have on your transcripts (time away from school)

Note: Do **not** include anything in your application that you are not willing to discuss at an interview. **Do** seek the counsel of your mentors on how to approach areas of weakness or special circumstances that you need to or opt to address in your application

[a]Performance here will be vital to securing interviews

12.2.1 General Surgery

General surgery offers a surgeon the opportunity of broad based training. It covers the essential practice of surgery, and is a required residency before pursuing additional training for many surgical subspecialties (It should be noted that an increasing number of surgical subspecialties now have integrated tracts, where training is matched into directly out of medical school; integrated training residencies are further addressed below, and in more detail in Chap. 12). Specialties requiring general surgery training prior to fellowship include, pediatric surgery, surgical oncology, endocrine surgery, colorectal surgery, minimally invasive surgery and hepatobiliary surgery among others. General surgeons are trained to manage and treat a wide spectrum of diseases across the entire body. A general surgeon has specialized knowledge about the: (1) the alimentary tract; (2) the abdomen & its contents; (3) breast, skin, and soft tissue; (4) head/neck, endocrine, congenital, and oncologic disorders; (5) the peripheral vasculature; (6) the endocrine system; (7) surgical oncology; (8) comprehensive management for trauma; and (9) complete care of critically ill patients with emergent surgical needs. General surgeons pride themselves on their broad surgical knowledge, the variety of procedures that they are able to perform, and their ability to address complex multi-system surgical issues. General surgeons have the opportunity to remain broad in their practice after training, may opt to narrow their scope of expertise with additional fellowship training, or may choose to focus on a specialty after their transition to practice.

General surgery training encompasses 5 years of clinical residency education within an accredited program. To become board certified in general surgery, the program must be accredited by specific organizations and The American Board of Surgery currently requires that a minimum of 750 operative procedures are completed, with 150 to be completed in the chief-resident year, although these requirements change often.[1] Many programs will require 1–2 years of research, which may take place after the 2nd post graduate year (PGY2) or third (PGY3) year and do not count towards the clinical training obligation.

Due to the broad training, diverse knowledge base, and multiple opportunities for further subspecialization, general surgery remains a cornerstone of the health system, with many residency positions (currently ~1,240 annually) offered in the National Resident Match Program.

12.2.2 Surgical Subspecialties

The following surgical specialties were traditionally subspecialties of general surgery and required completion of general surgery residency before continuing training in these areas. They now all offer 'integrated' positions where students match into the specialty directly from medical school in addition to the 'independent' tracks where training is entered after completion of general surgery residency. The

---

[1] http://www.absurgery.org/default.jsp?certgsqe_training

pros and cons of the different pathways are addressed in Chap. 12. For all of the integrated positions, students apply to programs just as they would for general surgery through ERAS and they are in the main residency match.

12.2.3 Plastic Surgery

According to the American Board of Plastic Surgery, a plastic surgeon deals with the "repair, reconstruction, or replacement of physical defects of form and function involving the skin and musculoskeletal systems". Plastic surgeons are able to address deformities and trauma related to craniomaxillofacial structures, hand, extremities, breast and trunk, external genitalia, and/or offer cosmetic enhancement to these areas of the body." Plastic surgeons have treatment expertise for a wide breadth of conditions and have considerable career flexibility. Plastic surgeons may choose to continue to further subspecialize in some of the following: craniomaxillofacial surgery, microvascular surgery, hand surgery, and cosmetic surgery. Outside of its broad and challenging technical demands, plastic surgeons have considerable flexibility in their choice of professional lifestyle, academic or professional practice, and research opportunities. As such, the field and practice of plastic surgery remains one of the constant innovators in surgery, and highlights the unique and exciting attributes of the profession.[2]

There are two different training pathways in plastic surgery: (1) an independent surgery program, which requires 3 years of training after the prerequisite general surgery requirement; and (2) the integrated program, that combines the prerequisite general surgery requirement and the training during the program's 6 year duration. Most commonly, an independent surgery program is entered into after completion of general surgery residency, although additional pathways include completion of training in other specialties such as: otolaryngology, neurosurgery, and oral-maxillofacial surgery.

Plastic surgery is a highly competitive surgical specialty. Traditionally, students applying for integrated position have been encouraged to apply to both general surgical training programs as well as plastic surgery programs due to the relatively small number of spots available. This is becoming less practical as general surgery has become more competitive in recent years, but it is still a strategy to consider.

12.2.4 Vascular Surgery

Vascular surgery is focused on the management and treatment of diseases of the vascular system. This includes surgical and non-surgical management of patients with these conditions. This specialty combines both open surgery and endovascular

---

[2] https://www.facs.org/education/resources/residency-search/specialties/plastic

treatment of vascular conditions. As such, training involves not only surgery but mastery of skills that include non-invasive vascular testing such as duplex ultrasonography, diagnostic angiography and therapeutic endovascular therapies. The evolution of this specialty combines many skill sets and offers the opportunity for a diverse practice. There are also multiple research opportunities in vascular surgery that include not only traditional translational science focused on vascular physiology, but diverse fields such as device development and testing. The independent pathway involves 2 years of training after completion of general surgery residency and most residents apply during their 4th year of residency. Integrated programs are 5 years in length and as noted are entered directly from medical school.

12.2.5   Cardiothoracic Surgery

Cardiothoracic surgery involves the care of diseases of the heart and chest (including the lungs, esophagus and mediastinum). Like other specialties, this has evolved from just open surgical management to include minimally invasive techniques for both cardiac and non-cardiac conditions. Most recently, there has been significant development in the fields of minimally invasive cardiac surgery that combines endovascular/interventional techniques with those of open surgery, and cardiac surgeons have led much of this effort. This has led to an expansion of the practice of cardiothoracic surgery and even greater opportunities for cardiac surgeons. As noted for other programs, the traditional, or independent, pathway to training involves completion of general surgery residency followed by 2 or 3 years (program dependent) of specialty training. The integrated programs for cardiothoracic surgery are 6 years in length and are matched into to out of medical school.

12.2.6   Surgical Specialties

The following surgical specialties are entered into directly from medical school. Historically, many trainees in these specialties completed 1 or 2 years of general surgical training as part of their program, but this has become less common. Urology and neurosurgery are 'early' programs in that the application process, and their respective applications move on a different timeline than the main residency match. These programs also participate in the the "San Francisco" match, which is separate from the National Residency Match Program.[3] Although this match functions similarly to the NRMP, it is completely separate from the main residency match.

---

[3] https://www.sfmatch.org/

12.2.7 Urologic Surgery

Urologic surgery or Urology is focused on the clinical diagnosis, medical and surgical management, prevention, and treatment of urologic diseases, neoplasms, deformities, disorders and injuries. Specialists in this discipline demonstrate knowledge and skill in the medical sciences relevant to the male genitourinary tract, the female urinary tract, and the adrenal glands. Urologists investigate infertility and male sexual dysfunction, as well as well as manage patients with structural and functional disorders of the kidney, ureter, bladder, prostate, urethra and male genitalia.

Urology residency programs match outside of the NRMP and participate in the American Urological Association (AUA Match). Urology residencies are considered one of the "early match" programs, which means that the application process is usually completed in late January, or about 6 weeks prior to the NRMP. Urology is regularly regarded as one of the most competitive surgical subspecialties, and thus applicants must excel in all domains of the ERAS application, along with strong letters of support. Sub-Internship is highly encouraged or required. Training requires 5 years of postgraduate education.

12.2.8 Neurological Surgery

Neurological surgery (often referred to as neurosurgery) manages disorders of the central and autonomic nervous systems, including their supporting systems and vascular supply. Neurosurgeons manage a wide variety of disorders affecting the brain, the spinal cord, spinal column, peripheral nerves, and extra-cranial cerebrovascular systems.

Neurosurgery residencies are usually between 6 and 8 years, including the intern year. The sequence of training usually follows the pattern: 1 year of internships; 1–2 years as a junior resident; 1 year as a mid-level resident; 1–2 years of protected research time or sub-specialty of your choosing, and finally 1 year as a chief resident.

All approved neurosurgical programs participate in the Neurosurgery Match Program. Neurosurgery participates in the "early match", and thus senior applicants are often encouraged to apply to both general surgical training programs as well as neurosurgery programs due to the minimal spots available. This is less common today as most applicants are not interested in both specialties. Preliminary years and substantial research experience are encouraged.

12.2.9　Orthopaedic Surgery

Orthopaedic surgery involves surgery of the musculoskeletal system. The scope of this specialty incorporates surgical and nonsurgical methodologies to prevent, investigate, diagnose, and treat disorders and injuries of the muscular and skeletal systems.

Orthopaedic surgery requires 5 years of graduate medical education and offers graduates a wide variety of subspecialties after residency completion including spine surgery, hand surgery, sports medicine, total joint replacement, pediatric orthopaedics, foot and ankle, and orthopedic oncology. This residency is noted for being highly competitive.

12.2.10　Otolaryngology: Head and Neck Surgery

Often referred to as an Ear, Nose and Throat (ENT) specialist, otolaryngologist-head and neck surgeon provides care for patients with conditions affecting the ears and upper aero-digestive systems that are related to the head and neck. This is a very diverse specialty that involves both surgical and non-surgical management of these conditions. Surgical care spans a broad spectrum including smaller office-based procedures to major cancer resections of the head and neck. This practice allows for a wide variety of practice settings with some otolaryngologists choosing to have a primarily office-based practice. In addition to general residency training, this specialty has a number of subspecialties and many trainees will choose to complete a fellowship for more focused training. Otolaryngology is highly competitive specialty that encompasses 5 years of clinical training. Most students successfully pursuing this specialty will have an excellent academic record.

12.3　What Programs Should I Apply To?

First, make sure that you want to become as surgeon. Review your motivations. Make sure that you have the field correctly assigned, as some procedures, and even surgical fields, are not considered surgical matches, ie. Gastroenterology, gynecological surgery or interventional radiology. The ability to perform procedures is not what defines a surgeon. It is imperative that you begin your journey in surgery very aware of the distinction between surgery and other specialties that have some procedural overlap, as the demands of the specialties are very different beginning with your 1st day of residency.

Once you decide upon your specialty, the process is similar to other academic applications that you have completed. A checklist can be used as a guide to help stimulate your thoughts on the decision to become a surgeon and your candidacy

☐ Know yourself – Are you really a surgeon?
☐ Strong qualifications
    ○ History of excellence including pre-medical school experiences
    ○ Grades
    ○ Boards
    ○ Evaluations
    ○ Letters of recommendation
        ▪ From your specific field of interest
            ▪ People who know you well
            ▪ People who think highly of you
            ▪ People who are highly regarded in the field
            ▪ People who have witnessed or supervised your clinical work
            ▪ Your chairman
☐ Commitment to the surgical field of your choice e.g. general surgery
    ○ Rotations
    ○ Related extracurricular activities
    ○ Research
    ○ Clubs
    ○ Travel
☐ Leadership potential
    ○ Research
    ○ Clubs
    ○ Travel
☐ Demonstrate a clear understanding of the required commitment
☐ Practice interviews with a mentor
☐ Devise a strategy to honestly address any gaps or inconsistencies in your application
☐ Enjoy the process, It is a Match!

Fig. 12.1 Checklist for a successful match into surgery – "Know your brand – Know your story"

(Fig. 12.1). It is helpful to map out your motivations and reasons for pursuing a particular area of surgery in addition to learning about the competitiveness of your candidacy prior to considering programs.

Ultimately, you must decide on the type of surgery that interests you in order to be competitive. Remember, surgery is just surgery to nonsurgeons; but to surgeons, the world of surgery is vast and wide. The type of operation, the level of intervention, and the patient population you serve are just a few of the major differences between surgical subspecialties. Personality types and attitudes and behaviors differ across people interested in different types of surgery and you want to be sure that you can demonstrate that you belong. Moreover, this is a big decision for you and it is important that you find a field in which you belong!

By now, hopefully you have a clear idea of how important the choice of residency will be for your medical career. The following questions outline a few things you may want to consider in your decision-making process:

1. What do I find most rewarding about surgery?
2. Will my choices within surgery allow me to utilize the skills that best suit me?
3. Will my choice incorporate the things that I find exciting about medicine and surgery?

4. What will my life look like during and after training? How much time will I devote to my career? Are there other personal life goals I have to consider?
5. Does financial opportunity and debt load impact my career choices?
6. What region of the country should I consider?
7. Do I want a big program or a smaller program? Urban or rural?
8. Am I interested in research? Quality improvement? Business of health care?

These questions should help you to narrow down the list of programs that you consider. Confide in mentors, your family, and friends about any reservations that you have. Make sure that your decisions are compatible with your best version of yourself. Be informed. Residency is a deeply personal decision, and no one will fault you for making the best decision for yourself. In fact, the reason the process is a "match", is to encourage a win-win for the applicant and the program, in that order!

Once you are certain of your decision and have decided which specialty fits you best, consider your competitiveness for both the specialty (as outlined above) and for individual programs. Resources for this include the individual web sites of programs you identify as interesting to you or have been suggested by your mentors. These often have key information that will be pertinent as you consider programs that best fit your application and career goals. Another resource is the Fellowship and Residency Electronic Interactive Database Access System (FREIDA) maintained by the American Medical Association (AMA).[4] This contains data populated by residency programs via an annual survey conducted jointly by the AMA and the Association of American Medical Colleges. This can help give you background information about individual programs.

12.4 How the Match Works

12.4.1 Electronic Residency Application System (ERAS)

The Electronic Residency Application System (ERAS) is the single, generic application that houses your basic demographic information, your curriculum vitae, your personal statement, letters of recommendation, USMLE Transcripts, and a list of the programs to which you are applying.[5] ERAS is the main application that will be sent to all of your selected residency programs. Program directors use the ERAS application to determine your competitiveness and utilize this interface to decide who will be invited for an interview. You can begin to edit your application in May

---

[4] http://www.ama-assn.org/ama/pub/education-careers/graduate-medical-education/freida-online.page
[5] https://students-residents.aamc.org/attending-medical-school/how-apply-residency-positions/applying-residencies-eras/

of the application year, and should plan to submit the application mid-September. You want to be complete on the day the system opens or certainly as early as possible. You can provide updates to your application over time. Do not worry about the Dean's letter as these seem to go in later and later each year. But, make sure to give your letter of recommendation writers plenty of advanced notice and reminders as the deadline approaches.

12.4.2 National Residency Matching Program (NRMP)

The National Residency Matching Program (NRMP) runs the main residency match that connects applicants with residency programs. (http://www.nrmp.org/) All residency programs registered in by the NRMP are accredited by the Accreditation Council on Graduate Medical Education. All applicants and participating institutions participate in the NRMP in the same fashion i.e. both applicants and programs rank each other, and the algorithm "matches" the highest ranked overlap of both applicant preference and program acceptance. No opportunity exists for either applicant or program to offer or accept an early position outside of the match.

Each applicant submits a Rank Order List. Each program submits an ordered list of interviewed applicants. Once the applicant has been "matched" to the highest ranked position on their list, the Match for that applicant then becomes final, and his/her name is removed from the list of all other programs. It is not possible to match in a lower ranked program, if you are slotted into a position at a higher ranked program on your list.

Urological surgery and neurosurgery do not participate in the NRMP match. As noted earlier, candidates for residency positions in these surgical subspecialties participate in a separate early match (San Francisco match). It is important for students interested in these specialties to check the timelines for the early match with their medical schools.

12.4.2.1 How Does the Couples Match Work?

The NRMP Registration, Rankings and Results (R3) system allows couples to participate in the Match as a pair. (http://www.nrmp.org/match-process/couples-in-the-match/) The system is designed to link rank lists at the request of a pair of applicants. Each person in the pair must enroll in the same Match, and indicate in the R3 system that he/she intends to participate as a pair. The individuals in the pair will need to rank the same combinations of programs. The match algorithm will treat the individuals as a pair. This will require a lot of discussions about preferences and competitiveness between the couple.

The couple's match works like the individual match in that coupled applicants will match at the highest rank combination in which both have been accepted. No formal documentation is needed to confirm the nature of the relationship between the pair to participate in the couple match; any two people may agree to pair within the match.

In 2013, couples matched with a 95.2 % success rate. This means that the system was able to identify a match that satisfied one of the combinations submitted by the pair. It does not mean that each member of the couple was as successful as they might have been individually. This process highlights the need for medical couples to compromise in order to achieve happiness in both personal and professional endeavors. The Couples Match does not extend to the Military Match or the early match. Couples entering into the couples match should discuss ranking options with their medical school advisors.

12.4.2.2 Military Match

The Military Match is for students who have been supported by the military's Health Professions Scholarship Programs (HPSP).[6] In exchange for financial support of a medical education, some students will complete residency training at a military hospital. Other students will have the option to request civilian deferment to complete residency at private institutions. It is encouraged that students enter both the Military Match as well as the NRMP, as those not selected for military GME still have time to apply and be successful.

12.4.3 Categorical and Preliminary Surgery Programs

A "categorical" residency program provides training for the requisite number of years and experiences required to become board eligible in a medical specialty. A "preliminary" surgery program is a basic entry position in a surgical program. Designated preliminary programs serve as transitional programs for people entering categorical programs that require 1 year of residency prior to enrollment in the program. Non-designated preliminary programs serve as a launching pad to a career in one of several specialties for people who do not match into categorical programs. Non-designated preliminary surgery programs can be used as an opportunity to improve an applicant's application and overall qualifications for the next year's residency match. They can also be used as an audition for a categorical spot at the sponsor institution for outstanding candidates.

---

[6] http://www.militarygme.org

12.4.4 Not Matching and the Supplemental Offer and Acceptance Program® (SOAP®)

Not everyone matches. Unmatched and partially matched applicants are notified a few days before the actual match, and encouraged to enroll in the SOAP (Supplemental Offer and Acceptance Program). (http://www.nrmp.org/residency/soap/) There is not a lot of time to recover from the emotional toll of not matching before the student needs to make meaningful decisions about his/her next step. If you do not match, you should call mentors and the guidance office at the medical school to fully and quickly explore options. The student must candidly review the application process, and future goals and objectives. There are five decisions to consider: (1) withdraw from the match and defer graduation to get a degree or do research to enhance the application for the following year, (2) enter the SOAP in the original specialty, (3) enter the SOAP for a different specialty, (4) graduate and choose an alternative career, or enter the match independently. The fourth choice is not recommended. At 6:00 pm (Eastern Standard Time) on the Thursday of Match week, a list of programs participating in the SOAP is made available through medical schools. All programs with unfilled spots can opt to participate.

Students can apply to the unfilled programs by submitting their ERAS application to the unfilled programs. They can submit applications to multiple specialties as well. Based upon the ERAS applications received, program directors create a preference list of applicants and positions are filled over the course of several application cycles. Applicants may receive multiple offers in any round; however, they have only 2 h to accept or reject an offer. The process continues until remaining programs are filled.

12.5 Conclusions

Your candidacy as a surgical resident depends upon your performance before and during medical school, as well as the specialty to which you are applying. You should be mindful of the characteristics of the successful applicant: honesty, integrity, hard-working and a committment to a surgical career. Use the provided tools to help assemble the pieces of your application. There are many paths to becoming a successful surgeon. You should find the path and location that will afford you the luxury of support and rigorous training. Embrace a career that will keep you engaged throughout your residency and beyond. Have fun and Good luck!

References and Helpful Links

General Surgery

https://www.facs.org/education/resources/residency-search/specialties/general

Plastic Surgery

https://www.abplasticsurgery.org/about-us/plastic-surgery/
https://www.facs.org/education/resources/residency-search/specialties/plastic

Vascular Surgery

https://vascular.org/career-tools-training

Cardiothoracic Surgery

http://www.sts.org/residents-students
http://www.tsranet.org/
http://www.ctsnet.org/program-profiles

Urology

https://www.facs.org/education/resources/residency-search/specialties/urology
https://www.auanet.org/education/urology-and-specialty-matches.cfm

Neurosurgery

https://www.facs.org/education/resources/residency-search/specialties/neuro
http://www.aans.org/Young%20Neurosurgeons/Medical%20Students/Questions%20You%20
   Should%20Ask.aspx

Orthopedic Surgery

https://www.facs.org/education/resources/residency-search/specialties/ortho
http://www.aaos.org/Membership/MedicalStudentResources/

Otolaryngology: Head and Neck Surgery

https://www.facs.org/education/resources/residency-search/specialties/oto
http://www.entnet.org/content/what-otolaryngologist

ERAS, NRMP and SF Match

https://www.aamc.org/services/eras/
http://www.nrmp.org/
https://www.sfmatch.org/

Chapter 13
The Application Process

Rishindra M. Reddy

Abstract The application process begins during the first and second years of medical school. Ultimately, all information in your CV, personal statement, letters of recommendation, and clinical clerkships will determine your ability to match into a residency program. Here we review the steps in the application process and the application itself with suggestions on how to maximize your chances of matching into a surgical residency. The recommendations in this chapter are based on students in a 4-year program, who complete their core clinical year during the 3rd year. Adjust the timeline based on your specific educational plan.

13.1 Introduction

Students must network with faculty surgeons for guidance and mentorship with the goal of making good career and life choices. Time spent preparing/studying for USMLE Step 1 and for your clinical clerkships is of critical importance as this will affect your application as much as any letters or personal statements or achievements. Later in the application process, it is important to concentrate efforts on the portions of the application that can be controlled – the CV, personal statement, letters of recommendation, and any remaining clinical clerkships. Once you've decided to pursue a career in surgery, or any field, start preparing your resume and thinking about your personal statement, while also considering which faculty to ask for letters of recommendation. It is imperative that your entire application is completed on time and ready for submission on the 1st day the application opens. Residency programs offer interviews on a rolling basis and you must check your email regularly to accept offers, as spots may fill up despite an offer to interview. The process is stressful for all students, whether you are applying to general surgery, pediatrics, or radiology, but early preparation and mentorship will help. The recommendations in

R.M. Reddy (✉)
University of Michigan, Ann Arbor, MI, USA
e-mail: reddyrm@med.umich.edu

© Springer International Publishing Switzerland 2017
M.J. Englesbe, M.O. Meyers (eds.), *A How To Guide For Medical Students,
Success in Academic Surgery*, DOI 10.1007/978-3-319-42897-0_13

this chapter are based on students in a 4-year program, who complete their core clinical year during the 3rd year. Adjust the timeline based on your specific educational plan.

Checklist for Application
[]-Curriculum Vitae (CV)/Resume
[]-Personal Statement
[]-Chair Letter of Recommendation
[]-Faculty Letters of Recommendation (2–3)
[]-Deans Letter
[]-USMLE Step 2

Checklist for Applicants in Preparation for Applying
[]-Schedule USMLE Step 2 if needed so that your scores will be back by September 15th
[]-Identify 2–3 mentors in the field (Clerkship Director, Faculty from Clinical rotations, etc)
[]-Meet with Chair to review CV and Personal Statement
[]-Meet with other mentors to review CV, Personal Statement, List of Residency Programs, etc.
[]-Solicit advice from resident mentors you have worked with
[]-Evaluate your personal web presence and address/eliminate any concerning information online
[]-Identify regional and/or urban preferences that you and/or your family have for residency
[]-Identify programs within your geographic preferences based on your interests and competitiveness (as deemed by mentors/clerkship director/chair).

13.2   Curriculum Vitae

Update your CV on a regular basis. You will need to do this for the rest of your professional life. It is hard to remember what you volunteered for 2 years ago during your preclinical education. As you near the completion of your M3 year, begin to review your CV and add anything that you think is relevant, including all educational activities, volunteer activities, etc. This can be trimmed later, but having everything possible included is the best starting point. An important consideration is how much undergraduate and high school activities to include. For your residency application, eliminate volunteer activities from these time periods unless they've had a significant influence/impact on you. Your serving as a tutor for elementary students as high school junior is irrelevant, and decreases the impact of more recent activities during your medical education. You also want to eliminate duplicates as some applicants list a presentation under both "Research" and "Abstract/Presentation" categories. The list of categories outlined below have been taken from a University CV template and sections that do not pertain to you should be deleted.

Education and Training This is a list of your university/college education, medical school, and any other graduate training with the date of degree given. Grade point averages, your "major", and any specific honors (Cum Laude, etc.) are included here. You should eliminate your high school unless there is something special that you want to highlight. Any special "Fellowships" may be included here if there is a specific education curriculum.

Certification and Licenses This may be less applicable at this stage in your life, but if you've completed Basic Life Support (BLS) training or other relevant certifications are included here.

Work Experience This may or may not have any content depending on your past history. Any relevant work experience that is important to you could be included. Part time work that you may have done when while in high school is not as relevant.

Research/Grants Here you can summarize your research experiences. Include a "title" of your research experience, the principle investigator (PI) or mentor, and the timeline of when this was completed. You may include a 1–2 sentence summary of the research and list any specific skills gained (western blots, statistical analysis, etc.). If you've received any research grants for summer research, etc., this would be a place to include that information also.

Awards and Achievements This includes the relevant awards and honors that you've received through your career and may include non-medical awards that reflect your strengths. Awards prior to your undergraduate education may be included if they are relevant and something that you feel should be highlighted for faculty/programs reviewing your CV.

Professional Society Memberships This section may be empty at first, but you may join professional societies once you've determined your long-term career interest. Many, if not all, professional societies will have candidate memberships that offer heavily discounted fees, but allow you free access to journals and possible educational materials. Joining these societies may allow you to find other mentors within the field. The American College of Surgeons offers a student membership with resources targeted at medical students that are valuable for students interested in surgery.

Committee/Volunteer Service Service in student government, student organizations, school-wide committees during medical school are included here, including the listing of specific leadership roles. Service in national organizations (AMSA, AMA, etc.) may also be included here. Undergraduate activities can be included here, on a more selective basis, by considering the value it adds to your application. If you clutter this area of the application, people will likely miss the substantive work you have done.

Invited Presentations There is often confusion on what is included in this field. School presentations that are part of the normal curriculum are NOT invited presentations. Seek help from faculty if you are unclear as to what include in this section, but some students add "talks" here that again dilute the importance of any real presentations.

Abstracts/Posters/Presentations Work resulting from specific research experiences can and should be listed here. For a student CV, it is OK to list internal (school specific forums/research days) and external (Clinical Congress, American College of Surgeons) presentations here. Highlight your name within the list of authors and list items chronologically. At the end you may state "This was a podium presentation at XXX meeting, or This was a poster presentation at XXX meeting". A presentation for research is DIFFERENT than an invited presentation in the previous category. Having a faculty review this portion of your CV may help. It is OK to list items if the abstract has been submitted, although this would not be acceptable on a faculty level CV.

Manuscripts Work from research, even if the presentation is listed above, is listed here. Subgroups may be listed if pertinent (Peer-Reviewed, Non-Peer Reviewed, Book Chapters). Again, highlight your name within the list of authors and list items chronologically. It is OK to list items if the paper has been submitted, although again this would not be acceptable on a faculty level CV. Note the status of the submission at the end (Submitted, Accepted, In press).

Media This is an area of evolution. If you have published material online that you would like to highlight, please include this. As stated above, take steps to review your online presence in social media and on the web in general – "Google" yourself. Please realize that if you cite something here, or if some of your work is searchable online, the program may form opinions about you based on that work.

Hobbies This is an area that allows you to list other important aspects to your life. Be specific but be concise.

13.3 Personal Statement

The personal statement can be one of the most important pieces of your application. It gives the reader some insight into who you are and who you want to be. You must be careful though about being too emphatic. Five percent of personal statements are works of literature, 80 % are bland but adequate, and 15 % are arrogant or odd. It is hard to be in that 5 %, and writing something that is meant to be humorous may come off as odd. The use of melodrama or "surgical anecdotes" will be off-putting to some readers. Your personal statement needs to include the following topics:

1. Why do you want to be a surgeon?
2. What makes you unique? Why should the program offer you an interview?

3. What are you looking for in a training program?
4. What are your long-term career goals?

It may be hard to think of ways to answer these succinctly, but there is a one page, single-spaced, length limitation. For the long-term career goals, think of a mentor or surgeon you know, who you want to emulate and describe that person. That may be easier than describing a new career path. Many surgeons respond well to athletic or musical experiences that required repetitive practice that can me related to surgery.

Chair Letter of Recommendation This is an important letter, but is often viewed just as a formality resulting in an impersonal letter with limited insight. Counteract this by getting to know the Chair through at least one in person meeting where you have your CV and draft personal statement available for review. You must convey your reasons for going into surgery and your long-term goals such that your Chair can include this in their letter. Having as much information as possible for the initial meeting will help your Chair. For many, the Chair may be a primary mentor, but that person can't serve that role for all students, and as such, your office meeting is of critical importance. The better prepared you are for that meeting, the more informative the Chair letter can be. Schedule a meeting with the Chair 2–3 months in advance of the application deadline, so that you can also get advice on programs, based on your regional and clinical interests. Prepare for this meeting by knowing the answer to the questions outlined above in the personal statement section. Be ready with questions of your own for the Chair.

Faculty Letters of Recommendation (2–3) These are from surgeons in the field you are applying to with few exceptions. Some medical schools have suggested that physicians from different specialties can write you letters. Be wary of this approach in the surgical specialties. Non-surgeons may write you a letter only if they know some aspect of your clinical/research background that would be relevant to your long-term career. Usually, only research mentors would fall into this category. No matter how well an internal medicine faculty knows you, it's not considered relevant for your surgery application. Finding letter writers may be difficult if you're not preparing for it early. If you know you are pursuing a career in surgery, mention the letter while you are rotating with that particular faculty mentor. These meeting could be as early as spring of M3 year but more often come during, or after, sub-internships. Have a draft of your CV and personal statement with questions about surgery residency, surgery lifestyle, and surgery programs. Most faculty at academic programs enjoy these meetings and look forward to giving you advice. Not utilizing faculty for advice is the most common made by medical students

Create an agenda for your first meeting to discuss with the faculty, and provide that agenda to them in advance. Review every aspect of your application and residency selection based on your individual academic performance. Take the information you get from each person with a grain of salt. Understand that each person has different experiences and different biases. Getting input from 3–4 people, including residents who have just gone through this process is essential. When you meet with the faculty, be clear that your goal is to obtain a letter of recommendation. Ask the faculty if they feel comfortable writing a "strong" letter. More experienced faculty should tell you if they can't write a strong letter for you. The worst part of your application could be a letter of recommendation that is written by someone who barely knows you. This may be a red flag for program directors, regardless of the prominence of the letter writer. Your letter writers help supplement your personal statement and CV by providing more context to areas that you want to highlight. For example, if a student has done research but has no publications, the research mentor may comment on the 4–5 manuscripts in preparation. Also, a letter writer can highlight special attributes that add depth to the applicant. Sharing this information with your faculty mentors, or discussing this during these meetings will be helpful. Multiple meetings may be required. They can be short but by maintaining a continued presence will facilitate a better letter.

Deans Letter This letter is a standard letter, also called the Medical School Performance Evaluation (MSPE), written by your Dean's office that includes your Preclinical and Clinical grades, along with information of where you fall within your class (i.e. top 25th percentile). This letter also includes information on the way that your medical school assigns grades at every level. This letter will be used going forward for fellowship applications in the future, and sometimes also for medical licenses and hospital credentialing. Most programs do not look at this in detail.

USMLE Step 2 There is no consensus on when to take Step 2. It is less important than Step 1, but if you have suboptimal Step 1 scores, taking Step 2 early and doing well helps your application. Your school may have specific criteria on when to take Step 2, so please be aware of this as you plan your M4 year. Students often reflect that taking Step 2 sooner, closer to completing the Core Clinical year, helps in doing better on the exam.

13.4 Timeline

The timeline for residency applications is posted on the American Association of Medical Colleges (AAMC) website. There may be minor variations each year.

Late May to early June ERAS (the Electronic Residency Application System) begins. Students can register on MyERAS and begin work on their applications. Letter of Recommendation Portal (LoRP) opens for authors to upload letters.

September 15 Applicants can submit their applications to ACGME-accredited programs. Residency programs then receive your application, with the exception of the MSPE (see below). YOUR APPLICATIONS SHOULD BE COMPLETE BY THIS DATE WITH LETTERS OF RECOMMENDATION.

October 1 MSPEs are released from your medical school Dean's office to residency programs.

September 15-Nov 1 This is when the majority of interviews are offered. Many students get an interview or 2 just days after submitting the application. This will peak during the first 2 weeks of October and tail off towards November. Occasionally, an applicant will be offered an interview position from a cancelled applicant later than November, but this is not universal for all applicants. Close attention to your email is critical to solidifying these interviews. Positions fill quickly, sometimes within an hour or less, and there may only be 1 or 2 days that will fit into your schedule. Once those days are filled, it is difficult to get a program to open an additional spot. If you are not hearing from some programs by early October seek out your mentors for further guidance.

October-February Interview season.

February Ranks lists are due from applicants and programs (Date changes each year).

March Match results are available during "Match week". On Monday, applicants will find out if they've matched to a program, though they won't know which program. The Supplemental Offer and Acceptance Program (SOAP, previous version was called the "Scramble") begins on Monday when those applicants who have not matched may begin contacting programs with open spots. This is coordinated through your medical school and should not be done on your own.

13.5   Conclusions

The application process begins as soon as you've decided on a career in surgery, by networking with faculty, studying for your Clerkship exams, and revising your CV. Input from mentors is critical on every aspect of the application process as outlined above, and all faculty are aware of the help that you need. There should be no surprise that you will need a letter of recommendation by September, so please be assertive in asking. Prepare for your faculty and chair advisory meetings with your CV, draft personal statement, and questions of your own. Submit your application on September 15th. Early preparation is essential. Faculty are seasoned veterans in this process; seek out their mentorship and guidance frequently throughout the process. With the proper work and mentor guidance, you can put yourself into an excellent place to match.

Chapter 14
Integrated Cardiothoracic Residency Programs: Pros and Cons

Jason P. Glotzbach and Scott C. DeRoo

Abstract This chapter focuses on training pathways for cardiothoracic surgery and the pros and cons of traditional pathways, where trainees enter the specialty after completing general surgery residency, and integrated tracks where students match directly into cardiothoracic surgery out of medical school. We will examine why one pathway might be best for you as an individual, but want to emphasize that both pathways lead to successful training and a fruitful career and there is not one 'best' way to pursue cardiothoracic surgery.

14.1 Introduction

Cardiothoracic surgery represents a vast field ranging from the treatment of thoracic malignancies and structural issues to the management of cardiovascular disease. Training is broad and demanding as patients are often older with multiple medical comorbidities. Despite the demands of a career in cardiothoracic surgery, it is a rewarding and engaging specialty unlike no other. Additionally, cardiothoracic surgery is changing and evolving such that the scope of practice is increasing. Although there has been concern in the past several years that the demand for cardiac surgeons is decreasing secondary to minimally invasive approaches, the opposite has proven true. As the number of interventional procedures has increased, the number of cardiac surgical procedures performed in the US has seen a concomitant increase

J.P. Glotzbach (✉)
Assistant Professor, Division of Cardiothoracic Surgery, University of Utah, Salt Lake City, UT, USA
e-mail: Jason.Glotzbach@hsc.utah.edu

S.C. DeRoo
Columbia University, New York, NY, USA
e-mail: Sd2857@cumc.columbia.edu

© Springer International Publishing Switzerland 2017
M.J. Englesbe, M.O. Meyers (eds.), *A How To Guide For Medical Students*, Success in Academic Surgery, DOI 10.1007/978-3-319-42897-0_14

likely due to improved detection of cardiovascular disease and updated guidelines recommending surgical management of patients with severe disease.

As a medical student considering potential career paths, one of the many factors that will inform your decision is the structure of the training paradigm for a given specialty. Given that cardiothoracic surgery remains one of the most demanding and challenging training paths one might choose, medical students considering a career in cardiothoracic surgery will naturally have many concerns regarding the training options in the modern era. The goal of this section is not to provide a detailed description of individual training programs or to advocate for one paradigm over another, but rather to provide a conceptual framework for medical students to understand the similarities and differences among the available cardiothoracic surgical training pathways. The authors offer the dual perspective of a "traditional" fellowship-trained CT surgeon who completed an entire general surgery residency before pursuing CT surgery training and an "I6" CT surgery resident currently completing an integrated cardiothoracic surgery residency program.

14.1.1 Training Program Structure

First, a word about terminology, traditional CT surgery training programs have traditionally labeled their trainees "residents," although colloquially they are often referred to as "fellows." A surgical fellow is technically a trainee that is pursuing advanced training in a field in which they have already completed core residency training. Although CT surgery trainees are often referred to as "fellows" in reference to their status as having completed general surgery training, CT surgery training represents a second residency rather than a subspecialty of general surgery (such as colorectal surgery).

The traditional training paradigm requires completion of a general surgery residency as a prerequisite before entering a cardiothoracic surgery residency program. Applicants typically apply for the CT surgery match during the fourth year of general surgery training, which allows for uninterrupted transition into CT training after completion of the general surgery chief residency year. Most fellowships will accept applicants into the CT surgery match with the assumption that they will complete general surgery residency training, but final admission to a CT surgery residency is not granted until the applicant has completed general surgery training. It is important to consider when selecting this pathway that during general surgery training you will be considered a general surgeon, not a future cardiothoracic surgeon. In most surgical training programs, there is minimal "elective" time and one typically cannot tailor the general surgery curriculum to reflect a specific interest towards a given sub-specialty such as cardiothoracic surgery. Some programs have developed a 4/3 model wherein a resident can start in general surgery but switch to CT surgery during the fourth year of residency and complete CT surgery training. This pathway may or may not allow for eligibility for the American Board of Surgery certification.

While a complete discussion of the general surgical residency training curriculum is beyond the scope of this chapter, it is important to consider that the exposure to cardiothoracic surgical services will vary among different general surgery residency programs. The American Board of Surgery requires experience in vascular surgery as part of general surgery residency, but does not explicitly require cardiovascular or general thoracic experience. Despite this lack of a formal requirement, many general surgery programs include rotations on the general thoracic service, in the cardiovascular or cardiothoracic intensive care unit, or even on the cardiac surgery service. In addition, trauma surgeons have historically been trained in thoracic trauma as part of their experience; therefore, general surgery programs that are strong in trauma will typically provide substantial exposure to thoracic trauma as part of the training curriculum. For students considering a "traditional" pathway of general surgery residency before CT surgery residency, it may be desirable to train in a general surgery program that provides some exposure to cardiovascular and thoracic surgery experiences during general surgery training.

CT surgery residency curriculums are organized into either a 2- or 3-year structure. The American Board of Thoracic Surgery stipulates that in order to become board eligible for Thoracic Surgery, one must complete training in general thoracic, adult cardiac and congenital cardiac surgery, including cardiovascular critical care (Thoracic Surgery Residency Requirements 2016). These rotations have expanded over the past decade to include additional training and experience in endovascular skills, interventional cardiology procedures, and mechanical circulatory support. Many residents elect to pursue advanced fellowship training in one of these areas following completion of CT surgery residency.

Current integrated cardiothoracic surgery programs are 6 clinical years in duration, often with an option for up to 2 years of dedicated research time. In general, the first 3 years are a combination of general and cardiothoracic surgical rotations, with several shorter duration rotations in cardiology, perfusion, echocardiography, and intensive care (Ward et al. 2013). The second 3 years are generally considered dedicated cardiothoracic surgery time, with a rotation schedule similar to traditional fellowship pathways. During the final 3 years of residency, integrated CT surgery residents assume a progressively more active role on the cardiac and thoracic surgical services.

Unlike other CT surgery training pathways, residents in integrated programs experience a mixture of general and CT surgery during their early training. While this does compromise the general surgery experience, it allows for increased exposure to cardiac and thoracic surgery throughout training. Cardiothoracic surgeons entering practice in the near future will need to be familiar with not only open cardiac surgery, but also minimally invasive techniques such as percutaneous valve replacement (TAVR), minimally invasive valve repair/replacement, and endovascular aortic repair (EVAR). Given the increasing scope of practice and diversity of procedures, it is beneficial to allow residents exposure to these techniques throughout their training. Conversely, many of the basic surgical skills necessary for cardiac surgery have traditionally been obtained through general surgical training. In decreasing resident exposure to general surgery, residents must acquire many of these skills on cardiac or thoracic surgical services, often in a higher acuity setting.

14.1.2   Advantages and Disadvantages of Integrated Cardiothoracic Training

In 2003, the American Board of Thoracic Surgery (ABTS) eliminated the requirement for American Board of Surgery certification for certification in thoracic surgery, which opened the door for the integrated pathway of thoracic surgery residency (Crawford 2005). Integrated cardiothoracic surgery training programs offer medical school students a pathway to begin their training immediately after medical school. This pathway has rapidly gained popularity over the past few years, and has become quite competitive (Varghese et al. 2014). As with all integrated surgical training pathways, there are advantages and disadvantages to choosing a surgical subspecialty without first completing a general surgery residency. Table 14.1 lists many of the pros and cons of an integrated surgical training program.

In general, integrated programs offer residents early exposure to their chosen specialty. Most, if not all, integrated cardiothoracic surgery training programs are designed to train individuals specializing in cardiac rather than thoracic surgery. As a result, there is often less emphasis placed on thoracic surgical education. In the current training environment, students who wish to pursue a career in general thoracic surgery should seriously consider the traditional training paradigm to receive the full benefit of general surgery training before focusing on thoracic surgery. As programs continue to evolve, many institutions may open designated thoracic track residency slots within the I6 program.

Table 14.1 Integrated surgery training

Pro	Con
Early exposure to surgical specialty	Need to choose sub-specialty in medical school
Shorter duration of training	Decreased opportunity for maturation and development during general surgery chief time
Longer time for development of mentorship relationship with surgical specialty faculty	Limited access to broader surgical faculty
Increased understanding and familiarity with surgical techniques of surgical specialty (particularly minimally invasive techniques)	Limited opportunity for mastery of basic surgical skills prior to focused (and often high-stress) specialty surgical environment
Ability to learn and become proficient in specialty over many years	Highly selective match
Ancillary rotations in affiliated fields more likely (e.g.- cardiology, ECHO and cardiac anesthesia in cardiothoracic surgery)	Decreased operative months
Increased focus on specific disease pathology	Lack of relevant general surgical training(e.g. foregut surgery for esophagectomy or abdominal surgery for open vascular surgery)
Increased time in area of interest	Not eligible for general surgery boards, if resident drops out would need to start over in general surgery or other specialty

If a medical student is relatively certain in the desire to become a cardiac surgeon, then the integrated program offers an unparalleled focus on cardiovascular disease throughout residency training. Conversely, the surgical foundation provided by a vigorous general surgery residency can be profoundly valuable in terms of technical development. If one does choose the traditional pathway, it is crucial to be fully committed to general surgery training. One potential pitfall is to "look past" the general surgery training. Such lack of engagement can sabotage your surgical training if you are not fully invested in becoming a proficient general surgeon first and proficient CT surgeon second. Medical students must be cognizant of this dynamic and not think of general surgery as a "backup" in case they are not successful in the integrated match. Some applicants applying to both integrated CT surgery and general surgery residency programs have reported a negative experience in general surgery interviews, likely as a result of a perceived decreased commitment to general surgery (Meza et al. 2015).

The integrated training model is relatively new to CT surgery, and as such only a handful of programs have produced graduates. Presently there does not appear to be a bias amongst potential employers in the academic or private sector with regard to hiring graduates of integrated training programs, but it is still very early in this paradigm. We expect that integrated programs will continue to mature and that graduates will be successful CT surgeons in diverse practice settings. However, the traditional training paradigm is a proven method for developing proficient cardiothoracic surgeons, and students should not feel pressure to choose the integrated pathway unless they are certain that CT surgery is the specialty they want to pursue. We expect both pathways to exist well into the near future. It is an exciting time for CT surgery and with the flexibility in training options; we are optimistic that an increasing number of medical students will choose to join this vibrant field.

References

Crawford Jr FA. Thoracic surgery education – past, present, and future. Ann Thorac Surg. 2005;79:S2232–7.

Meza JM, Rectenwald JE, Reddy RM. The bias against integrated thoracic surgery residency applicants during general surgery interviews. Ann Thorac Surg. 2015;99:1206–12.

Thoracic Surgery Residency Requirements. 2016. http://www.abts.org/root/home/certification/residency-requirements.aspx

Varghese Jr TK, Mokadam NA, Verrier ED, Wallyce D, Wood DE. Motivations and demographics of I-6 and traditional 5 + 2 cardiothoracic surgery resident applicants: insights from an academic training program. Ann Thorac Surg. 2014;98:877–83.

Ward ST, Smith D, Andrei AC, et al. Comparison of cardiothoracic training curricula: integrated six-year versus traditional programs. Ann Thorac Surg 2013;95:2051–4; discussion 4–6.

Chapter 15
Vascular Surgery Training: Multiple Pathways to Success

Katharine L. McGinigle and Jason Crowner

Abstract Much like in other surgical specialties, vascular surgery has more than one pathway to success. Alternate training pathways allow for individuals to choose which might be best for them and allow them to optimally accomplish their career goals. This chapter highlights the various vascular surgery programs and the pros and cons of each.

15.1 Introduction

In vascular surgery, there are three models of training to consider – the independent model of general surgery residency followed by vascular fellowship (5 + 2 pathway), early specialization programs (ESP) that in essence allow general surgery residents to begin their vascular training in what would have been their chief resident year (4 + 2 pathway), and the more recent integrated programs (0 + 5 pathway) (The American Board of Surgery 2016). While the American Board of Surgery no longer requires successful completion of the general surgery qualifying exam (written exam), those who are graduates of the independent or ESP pathways must have an approved application for the general surgery qualifying exam to assure they have met adequate case volume requirements for training. Correspondingly, the independent and ESP pathways both make it possible for trainees to be eligible for certification in both general surgery and vascular surgery. The integrated pathway allows for certification only in vascular surgery.

Pursuit of positions in the integrated program, like other integrated programs in thoracic and plastic surgery, is through the match as a medical student. The application process is administered through the Electronic Residency Application Service (ERAS) and the match through the National Resident Matching Program (NRMP). The independent pathway is pursued through the match during general surgery training with the match occurring in May, generally in the PGY 4 year of training. ESP programs began in 2003 and are limited in number; to date only ten vascular trainees have completed this pathway in six programs(Klingensmith et al. 2016).

K.L. McGinigle (✉) • J. Crowner
University of North Carolina, Chapel Hill, NC, USA
e-mail: Katharine_mcginigle@med.unc.edu; Jason_crowner@med.unc.edu

© Springer International Publishing Switzerland 2017
M.J. Englesbe, M.O. Meyers (eds.), *A How To Guide For Medical Students*,
Success in Academic Surgery, DOI 10.1007/978-3-319-42897-0_15

Since beginning in 2007 (with the first two 0 + 5 graduates in 2012), there has been a rapid increase in the number of integrated positions. In 2015, there were 57 integrated positions available in the match at 49 programs, a number that had risen from 30 available positions in the 2011 match (National Resident Matching Program 2015). In addition to the 57 integrated positions open in 2015, there were 115 positions available through the independent pathway at 90 programs. Those numbers have been essentially constant since 2011 (113 positions in 87 programs that year) (National Resident Matching Program 2015). Despite the increase in number of integrated positions over this time, it appears clear that the independent pathway will continue to be a viable and important way to pursue a career in vascular surgery and this is not expected to change.

The general pros and cons of integrated compared to traditional programs certainly applies to vascular surgery as well, but the data would suggest that both pathways produce positive training experiences (Dansey et al. 2016; Colvard et al. 2015). Similarly, in one early survey, it appears that the integrated pathway trainees are accepted by the surgical community, although some reservations existed about the maturity level and open operative skills of graduates (Kiguchi et al. 2014). It is not a surprise that integrated trainees perform far fewer "general surgery" cases during their training since it is 2 years shorter than traditional training (Smith et al. 2016). The overall fewer "general surgery" cases performed during training may impact surgeon experience at completion of training, but this seems to be offset by a far greater and longitudinal experience with vascular surgery and vascular diseases.

As noted above, despite several pathways to becoming a vascular surgeon, all roads lead to Rome and any of the approved paradigms will provide appropriate training for a career as a vascular specialist. A few considerations for you as a student considering a career in vascular surgery. First, if you are not sure whether vascular surgery is right for you, then general surgery followed by a vascular fellowship is the best career choice. This pathway gives you a breadth and depth of experience, allowing you to weigh each specialty and make a more informed career choice. The 5 + 2 pathway is not being phased out and is tried and true for launching a vascular surgery career. Second, if you are considering a career in vascular surgery and are leaning towards the integrated pathway, get involved as early as you can to confirm your choice. With decreasing overall exposure to surgery as a medical student, you will have a much better idea of whether the more direct, integrated pathway is right for you by spending time early on in your medical school career learning more about the specialty. Many medical schools have surgical interest groups and the Society for Vascular Surgery has developed resources for medical students as well (https://vascular.org/career-tools-training/develop-my-training-career).

There are many surgical specialties and many possible career paths within each, so it is important to ask many different kinds of surgeons what they like and don't like about their field. While it may seem daunting to approach many faculty surgeons, most will be happy to discuss their experiences with you. Additionally, the residents or fellows in training programs at your institution may also be a great resource. If vascular surgery still seems like an attractive career choice, then don't hesitate to take the relationship a step further and seek out a vascular surgery mentor at your institution. This will allow you to get involved in both clinical care and research opportunities. Finding mentors early in medical school can help you choose a specialty, and may also be important in helping you accomplish your career goals in the future.

References

Colvard B, Shames M, Schanzer A, Rectenwald J, Chaer R, Lee JT. A comparison of training experience, training satisfaction, and job search experiences between integrated vascular surgery residency and traditional vascular surgery fellowship graduates. Ann Vasc Surg. 2015;29(7):1333–8.

Dansey K, Wooster M, Shames M. Integrated vascular surgery resident satisfaction. Ann Vasc Surg. 2016;29(8):1581–8.

Kiguchi M, Leake A, Switzer G, Mitchell E, Makaroun M, Chaer RA. Perceptions of society for vascular surgery members and surgery department chairs of the integrated 0 + 5 vascular surgery training paradigm. J Surg Educ. 2014;71(5):716–25.

Klingensmith ME, Potts JR, Merrill WH, Eberlein TJ, Rhodes RS, Ashley SW, et al. Surgical training and the early specialization program: Analysis of a national program. J Am Coll Surg. 2016;222(4):410–6.

National Resident Matching Program. Results and data: 2015 main residency match. Washington, DC: National Resident Matching Program; 2015.

Smith BK, Kang PC, McAninch C, Leverson G, Sullivan S, Mitchell EL. 0 + 5 Vascular surgery residents' operative experience in general surgery: An analysis of operative logs from 12 integrated programs. J Surg Educ. 2016;73(3):536–41.

The American Board of Surgery. Pathways in vascular surgery.Training pathways. 2016. http://www.absurgery.org/default.jsp?certvsqe_primarycert

Chapter 16
Plastic Surgery Training in the Era of Integrated Programs

Michelle Roughton and C. Scott Hultman

Abstract Plastic surgery training has undergone and evolution in the recent past, like several other surgical specialties, and no longer follows the paradigm of surgical residency followed by specialty training. Although those traditional pathways exist, and allow for entry into plastic surgery from several specialties, integrated programs allow students to match into plastic surgery from medical school. This chapter examines both pathways and offers thoughts on how to be successful in pursuing training in plastic surgery.

16.1 Introduction

Traditional, independent plastic surgery training is 3 years long and most commonly follows completion of a full general surgery residency. However residents completing neurosurgery, otolaryngology, oral-maxillofacial surgery, orthopedics, and urology are also eligible for plastic surgery training (www.ACGME.org). Although commonly referred to as a 'fellowship', plastic surgery is truly a second residency and as such, residents are not allowed independent operating room privileges. Independent residents apply through the San Francisco match (https://www.sfmatch.org/).

Integrated plastic surgery residency is a 6-year training program where residents spend 3 or less years in general surgery and the remaining time in plastic surgery and related rotations. Like other integrated programs, this is an NRMP match from medical school.

M. Roughton (✉) • C.S. Hultman
University of North Carolina, Chapel Hill, NC, USA
e-mail: michelle_roughton@med.unc.edu; scott_hultman@med.unc.edu

The integrated plastic surgery match is competitive. In fact, with a 2014 match success rate of 72 % (up from previous years around 50 %), the integrated plastic surgery match is the most competitive of all medical specialties (www.nrmp.org). Many applicants apply to two specialties (most commonly general surgery) to increase their success rate in the match.

The integrated track is appealing to applicants as it takes less time to complete training. For some, this translates into increased freedom to pursue further subspecialty training available in craniofacial, aesthetics, hand, and microsurgery. For others, it is appealing to hone in on their chosen field earlier in their career rather than perfect many operations they will no longer perform.

The independent track also continues to thrive. Many medical students are not exposed to plastic surgery in their medical school curriculum and as such do not discover their aptitude or interest in the field until residency training. A common theme is the general surgery resident discovering breast reconstruction following mastectomy deciding their passion lies in "filling the hole, rather than making it." The independent track is less competitive than the integrated pathway allowing for applicants who may have built their resumes slightly later in training to pursue their chosen specialty.

Integrated and independent residencies have the same ACGME program educational requirements, i.e. case minimums, curriculum components, and milestone evaluations to ensure the production of competent well-rounded plastic surgeons. The integrated program additionally has core surgery minimum operative numbers for the early years (traditionally spent on general surgery services).

It is very likely that both tracks to plastic surgery will remain in place indefinitely. A driving factor for the continuation of the independent track is financial. Many academic divisions and departments must cover the cost of the resident salaries. This means that conversion to an integrated from an independent models doubles the cost (3–6 years) of training.

In summary, many factors are to be considered in the decision between integrated versus independent training in plastic and reconstructive surgery. The integrated match is competitive from medical school but does shorten the number of years to complete residency. The independent match, most commonly pursued after completion of general surgery, is less competitive but does take longer to complete. Both tracks have nearly identical curricula and produce qualified, capable, and competent plastic surgeons (Table 16.1).

Table 16.1 Integrated surgery training

Pro	Con
Early exposure to surgical specialty	Need to choose sub-specialty in medical school
Shorter duration of training	Decreased opportunity for maturation and development during general surgery chief time
Longer time for development of mentorship relationship with surgical specialty faculty	Limited access to broader surgical faculty
Increased understanding and familiarity with surgical techniques of surgical specialty (particularly specialty-specific techniques like microvascular surgery)	Limited opportunity for mastery of basic surgical skills prior to focused (and often high-stress) specialty surgical environment
Ability to learn and become proficient in specialty over many years	Highly selective match
Ancillary rotations in affiliated fields more likely	Decreased operative months
Increased focus on specific disease pathology	Lack of relevant general surgical training (e.g. breast or soft tissue surgery)
Increased time in area of interest	Not eligible for general surgery boards, if resident drops out would need to start over in general surgery or other specialty

References

https://www.sfmatch.org/. Accessed 16 Mar 2016.

www.ACGME.org. Accessed 16 Mar 2016.

www.nrmp.org. Summary statistics 2014. Accessed 16 Mar 2016.

Chapter 17
Choosing a Residency Program

Christiana Shaw and George A. Sarosi Jr.

Abstract After making the decision to pursue a career in surgery, the choice of a residency training program is likely to be the second most important professional decision you make. Where you go for residency plays a tremendous role in your future career. It can determine future productivity, practice type (academic or community), or even number of publications and success in academic medicine (Beninato et al. 2016; Campbell et al. 2011). Although the process of selecting the best residency seems incredibly daunting and complex, taking a systematic approach can make the process less difficult. So, as with most major decisions or journeys, you should begin with the end in mind.

17.1 Identify Your Goals

Spend some time thinking about both your personal and professional goals. Make a list of each, ranked by importance, and then integrate these two lists. Identify conflicts and opportunities. How will you manage the conflicts? How will you be best poised to achieve your goals? Take these items into consideration when selecting where to apply for residency.

There are many different career paths within the discipline of surgery, from a primarily outpatient community practice to a high-acuity tertiary referral center, part-time or full-time, rural, or urban. An important consideration as you define your goals is to consider how you want to spend your time as a surgeon. Are you interested in a career that is devoted mostly to providing clinical care, or are you interested in combining clinical surgery with other non-clinical pursuits such as research and/or surgical education? Do you have a strong interest in international medicine, public health, or medical administration? Many surgical subspecialties will require further training beyond your surgery residency in the form of a fellowship. If you are interested in one of these fields, general surgery residency is not the only educational consideration as greater than 70 % of residents pursue subspecialty fellowship training (Stitzenberg and Sheldon 2005).

C. Shaw (✉) • G.A. Sarosi Jr.
University of Florida, Gainesville, FL, USA
e-mail: Christiana.Shaw@surgery.ufl.edu; George.sarosi@surgery.ufl.edu

© Springer International Publishing Switzerland 2017
M.J. Englesbe, M.O. Meyers (eds.), *A How To Guide For Medical Students*,
Success in Academic Surgery, DOI 10.1007/978-3-319-42897-0_17

17.2   Understand Differences in Residency Programs

Understanding the different flavors of residency training programs is a key part of choosing your training program. There are currently 262 accredited residency programs in the United States (https://apps.acgme.org/ads/Public/Reports/ReportRun? ReportId=1&CurrentYear=2015&SpecialtyId=99&IncludePreAccreditation=false), most of which will offer high-quality training in surgery. Broadly, programs are described as one of two types, either university training programs or independent training programs. University training programs are tightly affiliated with a medical school in the United States. The primary hospital in the program is usually the major teaching hospital for the medical school and most of the surgeons in the training program have faculty appointments in the medical school. Surgeons at university training programs tend to have specialized, narrow practices and patients tend to be very complex. Total case volume at university programs tends to be lower, but residents in these programs tend to perform significant numbers of complex operations. These programs often have multiple post-residency fellowships. Independent training programs are not directly affiliated with one of the medical schools, although they may participate in medical student education. They are typically based in community hospitals, tend to expose residents to operative experiences early, and may not have the breadth of cases seen in university programs. Teaching surgeons in independent programs tend to be volunteer faculty and have more broad based practices than university surgeons. These programs often have fewer fellowships (Jones and Sidwell 2016).

Another factor students will want to consider is the presence of a research requirement or the ability to perform full-time research while a resident. About 35% of surgery residents will spend some additional time during their training engaged in full time research (Robertson et al. 2009). Twenty percent of surgery training programs have the majority of their residents spend time in full-time research with most of these residents taking 2 years of research. These research-intensive programs tend to be university based, and in many of these research is a required part of the training. For students who desire an academic career, or for those students who are planning on entering a competitive fellowship after general surgery (such as pediatric surgery or surgical oncology), the ability to perform research will be an important factor in choosing a residency.

The presence of clinical fellowships at a training institution is another factor to consider. Many training programs will also host post-residency fellowships in vascular, pediatric, colorectal, and minimally invasive surgery in addition to a general surgery program. This is more common in university training programs than independent programs. Roughly 75% of general surgery residents will choose to enter a fellowship at the conclusion of general surgery training (Klingensmith et al. 2015). The presence of clinical fellowships may be very helpful to residents interested in these fields because of increased availability of nationally recognized mentors. It may also allow residents an inside track to match at their home institution. However, the presence of clinical fellowships could reduce the resident operative experience in these areas, as residents and fellows may find themselves competing for cases. There is limited data to support this contention, but it remains a concern for many students (Hanks et al. 2011).

The size, location, and structure of a training program are also important factors to consider in choosing a training program. Programs can be divided into small (1–3 graduating chiefs per year), medium (4–5 chiefs per year), and large (6 or more chiefs per year). The structure of a training program typically refers to single hospital programs as compared to those programs where residents rotate through multiple hospitals, and the location of a program is typically urban or suburban compared with rural. Small programs may provide residents with more individual exposure to faculty and more personal attention, but may have less robust didactic programs. Small programs may be more affected by resident attrition, both in terms of the impact on remaining residents by the loss of one of their number and perhaps a higher crude attrition rate (Yeo et al. 2010). Large programs will likely have more robust educational infrastructure, and a larger faculty, but may suffer from less individual attention for residents. Urban training programs will typical serve a larger patient base, allowing for a greater diversity of patient experiences, but are often based in hospitals that function as safety net hospitals. These safety net hospitals often have fewer ancillary resources devoted to patient care and residents may have a higher burden of service activities such as clerical and patient transport duties. Single hospital training programs will require a resident to learn only a single electronic medical record system, and will likely increase clinical efficiency, but may limit exposure to specific patient populations, and will likely require away rotations in other health systems. Multi-hospital programs will likely require knowledge of multiple EMRs, may require significant commuting to hospitals in the system, which in an urban setting can be trying, and may cause issues of clinical efficiency related to switching between hospitals. They are however more likely to approach the ideal patient mix of a university hospital, a community hospital, a county or VA hospital, and a pediatric hospital in a single program. Away rotations for clinical experiences are rarely required in these programs.

17.3 Review Your Personal Strengths and Weaknesses

After gaining a better understanding of programs, take a critical look at your own application. Appreciate and understand differences in candidates, and your personal strengths and weaknesses. Every specialty will have certain criteria that are valued by program directors in selecting applicants to interview. For general surgery the top five characteristics are grades in required clerkships including the number of honors grades, USMLE Step I scores, quality of letters of recommendation, and membership in AOA (Alpha Omega Alpha) (Green et al. 2009). It is known that highly competitive programs are more likely to rank applicants with a history of prior research and publications, AOA membership, higher Step 1 scores, and excellent personal statements (Stain et al. 2013). Predictors of ranking by an independent residency program are slightly different and include USMLE scores, location of your medical school, and where you grew up. These programs tend to select candidates from specific regions of the country in line with their regional focus (Dort et al. 2015). Other non-academic factors that can effect your competitiveness include a history of high stakes competition, such as athletic or performance success, a history of substantive employment, or strong leadership experience either in medical school or before medical school.

17.4   Identify a Mentor

Prior to applying for surgery training, identify a mentor for the application process. Ideally this should occur in the last part of the third year of medical school. Mentors can help students with career plans, they can advise you on course selection in your fourth year of medical school, they can go over your curriculum vitae and identify areas for improvement, and may be able to help with residency applications. They may be able to introduce you to others in your chosen specialty. They may have opportunities for research, and may even consider you for awards or appointed leadership positions. One review of surgical mentors found the most frequently mentioned qualities of an effective mentor included serving as a professional role model and staying involved in terms of time and effort (Patel et al. 2011). Your primary mentor for your residency application process must be a surgeon, ideally one who is involved in the process of resident recruitment and selection. If you have another strong mentor in medical school from outside of surgery, this person can also be of assistance, but your surgical mentor will be key in your application process. Even if they are not selected as your mentor, your Clerkship Director, Program Director, or Chairman of Surgery at your home institution can help with the application process, and you must try to meet with him or her early in the application process. If you are unable to find a mentor at your home institution, consider the American College of Surgeons Young Fellow Association (https://www.facs.org/member-services/yfa/mentor), or the Association for Surgical Education (https://surgicaleducation.com/).

Once you identify a mentor, you will need to meet and discuss your career and training goals, and the details of your medical school performance and CV. One of the most important functions of your mentor is to carefully review the details of your academic and non-academic achievement and give you a realistic impression of your competitiveness for the surgery match. Not every future surgeon is a top applicant coming out of medical school. Many aspects of your application can make your competitive for surgery training, and grades and USMLE scores are only one facet of your application.

17.5   Create a List of Programs and Apply

The most important step in choosing your future training program is to identify the programs to which you will apply. In order to match in a training program you must interview and rank a program, and in order to interview you must apply and be selected to interview. Based on your career goals, your desires regarding where in the country you would like to train, and your review of your competetiveness for the match with your mentor you will need to build a list of programs where you will submit applications. A number of sources of information are available to help build your list of programs. These include web resources such as FRIEDA Online (http://www.ama-assn.org/ama/pub/education-careers/graduate-medical-education/freida-online.page) and the ACGME program search function (https://apps.acgme.org/ads/Public/Programs/Search). In addition, individual surgery program websites will contain a trove of information about each program. When looking at individual program websites, pay close attention to minimum USMLE scores and other requirements. Applying to programs where you do not meet the minimum requirements is unlikely to result in an interview.

A valuable source of current information about surgery training programs are the current surgery PGY-1 residents with whom you work. These resident have just been through the process you are starting and are a great source of data about differences in surgery training programs. Your surgical mentors can also help you build this list, but you should first review online and other sources before talking to them. Your mentor will be most valuable in helping you decide if the programs you have identified are ones where you will be competitive for an interview. Data from the National Resident Match Program (NRMP) shows that the median number of applications submitted by US Senior students who successfully matched is 42. This number of applications resulted in 18 interview invitations and 13 interviews attended (http://www.nrmp.org/wp-content/uploads/2016/04/Main-Match-Results-and-Data-2016.pdf). Interestingly this same data shows that applicants who did not match applied to more programs and received fewer interviews, suggesting that applying to more programs if you are not competitive will not improve your chances of interviewing or matching.

After you submit your applications for residency through the Electronic Residency Application Service (ERAS), programs will receive your application and make choices about offering interviews. There are a couple of important timeline considerations to remember. Applications are released to programs on September 15, and the Medical Student Performance Evaluations (Deans letter) are released to programs on October 1. Although the deadline for submitting an application is December, your application should be completed and submitted no later than October 1. Programs will begin to offer interviews in October and into November. Most programs will receive between 750 and 1000 applications and will offer 60–100 interviews based on these applications. It will take programs time to review applications, and just because the process is electronic, it is not instantaneous. Contacting programs you have not heard from prior to late October is not likely to increase you chances of getting an interview and should be avoided.

17.6 Identify the Interviews You Will Attend

Programs will contact you, most commonly through ERAS or by email, when they choose to offer you an interview, and this process occurs in a rolling fashion. When you are offered an interview you should contact the program rapidly to schedule the interview. Most programs will offer a few interview days only, and most are not flexible. Most interviews are offered between late October and late January. You should make sure that your fourth year medical school schedule offers you the flexibility to attend interviews. As you receive multiple interview offers you may develop scheduling conflicts that will prevent you from attending all of the interviews. Do not be concerned, as your goal is to attend between 12 and 14 interviews to have a high probability of matching. Interviewing is an expensive and time consuming proposition and you may not be able to attend all of the interviews you are offered. Your advisor can help you choose between programs and you should communicate with them as you choose which interviews to accept or reject. It is very important that if you accept an interview and then later choose not to attend the interview for whatever reason, that you contact the program as soon as possible to let them know of your choice. If you communicate promptly with the program they can offer this interview to another applicant. Holding on to interviews you will not attend is both inconsiderate to the program and may prevent another student from successfully matching!

17.7 Create Your Rank List and the Match

Immediately after interviewing at each program, write down specific aspects of the program you liked and disliked. Consider how these items factor into your long-term goals, and begin to assemble a rank list. Consider the differences among programs previously discussed: University vs. Independent, with or without a research requirement, presence or absence of fellowships, and size, location, and structure of the program. Again, meet with your mentor, Program Director, and/or Clerkship Director and discuss your rank list.

The match is a binding process, so only rank those programs where you would like to train. You will be expected to sign a contract for the position you are offered immediately following the results of the match. Also do not rank programs where you did not interview. Programs only rank candidates they interviewed, so no match will occur at programs where you did not interview.

The NRMP uses an algorithm to place applicants that is "applicant-proposing", meaning the preferences expressed on the rank order lists submitted by applicants (not programs), initiate placement into residency training. Therefore the applicant obtains the best possible outcome. The process begins with an attempt to match an applicant to the top choice program. If the applicant cannot be matched to that first choice program, an attempt is made to place the applicant into the second choice program, and so on, until the applicant obtains a tentative match or all choices have been exhausted. An applicant who is matched to a program may be removed from that program to make room for an applicant more preferred by the program. If an applicant is removed from a tentative match, an attempt is made to re-match that applicant, starting from the top of the applicant's rank list. More information can be found on the NRMP website, http://www.nrmp.org/match-process/match-algorithm/.

Changes can be made to your rank list until the deadline, but prior to consideration in the match, your list must be saved and certified. A list that is saved but not certified will not be eligible to match. Do not forget to certify your list on time!

17.8 If You Do Not Match

Your first opportunity to reapply is immediate – the SOAP (Supplemental Offer and Acceptance Program) happens during match week. For more information, visit the NRMP website: http://www.nrmp.org/residency/soap/. Following the SOAP, you may check the APDS (Association of Program Directors in Surgery) website for programs that remain or become unfilled: http://apds.org/education-careers/open-positions/.If you are unable to secure a position, strongly evaluate your application. Consider spending time in research or otherwise improving what is lacking in your application. Finally, reconsider surgery as a career choice. There are many exciting and worthwhile careers within medicine.

References

Beninato T, Kleiman DA, Zarnegar R, Fahey TJ 3rd. Can future academic surgeons be identified in the residency ranking process?. J Surg Educ. 2016;73(5):788–92.

Campbell PG, Lee YH, Bell RD, et al. Medical school and residency influence on choice of an academic career and academic productivity among US neurology faculty. Arch Neurol. 2011;68(8):999–1004.

Dort JM, Trickey AW, Kallies KJ, Joshi AR, Sidwell RA, Jarman BT. Applicant characteristics associated with selection for ranking at independent surgery residency programs. J Surg Educ. 2015;72(6):e123–9.

Green M, Jones P, Thomas Jr JX. Selection criteria for residency: results of a national program directors survey. Acad Med J Assoc Am Med Coll. 2009;84(3):362–7.

Hanks JB, Ashley SW, Mahvi DM, et al. Feast or famine? The variable impact of coexisting fellowships on general surgery resident operative volumes. Ann Surg. 2011;254(3):476–83; discussion 483–475.

https://apps.acgme.org/ads/Public/Reports/ReportRun?ReportId=1&CurrentYear=2015&SpecialtyId=99&IncludePreAccreditation=false. Accessed 20 May 2016.

Jones J, Sidwell RA. Residency surgical training at an independent academic medical center. Surg Clin North Am. 2016;96(1):147–53..

Klingensmith ME, Cogbill TH, Luchette F, et al. Factors influencing the decision of surgery residency graduates to pursue general surgery practice versus fellowship. Ann Surg. 2015;262(3):449–55; discussion 454–445.

Patel VM, Warren O, Ahmed K, et al. How can we build mentorship in surgeons of the future? ANZ J Surg. 2011;81(6):418–24.

Results of the 2015 NRMP apllicant survey by preferred specialty and applicant type. Washington, DC: National Resident Matching Program; 2015.

Robertson CM, Klingensmith ME, Coopersmith CM. Prevalence and cost of full-time research fellowships during general surgery residency. Ann Surg. 2009;250(2):352; author reply 352.

Stain SC, Hiatt JR, Ata A, et al. Characteristics of highly ranked applicants to general surgery residency programs. JAMA Surg. 2013;148(5):413–7.

Stitzenberg KB, Sheldon GF. Progressive specialization within general surgery: adding to the complexity of workforce planning. J Am Coll Surg. 2005;201(6):925–32.

Yeo H, Bucholz E, Ann Sosa J, et al. A national study of attrition in general surgery training: which residents leave and where do they go? Ann Surg. 2010;252(3):529–34; discussion 534–526.

Chapter 18
Perspectives of a Fourth Year Student

Jason Pradarelli

Abstract Many articles describe the dos and don'ts of interviewing for residency. While these tips are helpful for all residency applicants, there are nuances to consider when applying for surgery residencies that prioritize academic surgery. This chapter will focus on helping residency applicants stand out from the crowd and present themselves as exceptional candidates for top-tier academic surgery program.

It would be foolish to think that any outstanding applicant achieved their accomplishments on their own; mentors play an instrumental role in an applicant's competitiveness for residency programs through letters of recommendation and personal relationships with other programs. Once granted an interview, it is up to the applicant to put their best foot forward. The following advice will focus on helping residency applicants stand out from the crowd and present themselves as exceptional candidates for top-tier academic surgery programs.

18.1 What Academic Surgery Programs Want

In order for applicants to best sell themselves, it is important to understand what they are selling themselves for. The mission of academic surgery residency programs is to produce the future leaders in surgery. These programs desire to train surgeons who will go on to advance the field of surgery through their future careers. Surgeons may advance their field through discovery of new treatments for surgical

J. Pradarelli (✉)
Brigham and Women's Hospital, Boston, MA, USA
e-mail: jpradarelli@partners.org

© Springer International Publishing Switzerland 2017
M.J. Englesbe, M.O. Meyers (eds.), *A How To Guide For Medical Students*,
Success in Academic Surgery, DOI 10.1007/978-3-319-42897-0_18

diseases, improving surgical training, expanding surgical services to underserved patient populations, or countless other ways not yet imagined.

Applicants distinguish themselves by describing how they envision their career advancing the field of surgery. Although the written residency application supports potential for success, the interview is a time where key members of a residency program form initial impressions. The interview process offers a unique opportunity for applicants to advertise their strengths and passions and to present a convincing case that they will become leaders in surgery.

18.2 Interviewing with the Department Chair and Program Director

While all faculty members play an integral role in the department of surgery at a given institution, the department chair and program director are responsible for the quality, reputation, and culture of their residency program. These individuals have the most vested interests in residency candidates because the quality, reputation, and culture of a residency program are determined by the entirety of the department, including the residents. These residents will go on to represent their residency programs during their future careers.

With this in mind, applicants should be most prepared for interviews with these individual in a clear and convincing manner: *How will you make your impact in the field of surgery?* At academic surgery programs, this question will be asked to help department chairs and program directors determine if a candidate has potential to become a leader in surgery. Applicants should answer this question by building a strong case for *why* and *how* their story indicates that they will indeed change the world of surgery (or at least a part of it).

An effective way to build this case is to tell a story—a convincing story. While CVs and letters of recommendation list accomplishments, the interview offers an opportunity to tie all of these bullet points into a cohesive sales pitch. Applicants do not need to have a detailed, step-by-step plan for how they will transform the practice of surgery. However, any extra-curricular passion presented in the context of surgery can be a perfect theme around which to tell an applicant's story.

The response to this question should have a beginning, a middle, and an end. *How did this extra-curricular interest arise?* The applicant should start by explaining how they first acquired a passion outside of day-to-day clinical surgery. This could have happened through various experiences or projects worked on during medical school or through certain inspirational mentors encountered over the years. *How will the applicant cultivate this passion during residency?* This part of the story requires some work on behalf of the applicant. An applicant may search for faculty members at the interviewing institution who are working on projects that align with the applicant's passion. Identifying a connection with a faculty member's work—however vague the connections may be—is a strong bridge to an applicant's story. *How does the applicant envision this passion shaping their future career as a surgeon?* This portion should describe the applicant's vision for their future. In explaining how the applicant's passion will motivate their professional career, a cohesive story can come full circle and provide the punctuation for a convincing impression on the residency program's leadership.

By telling a story that integrates past accomplishments with underlying motivations and future goals, an applicant is perceived as more mature, credible, and poised for success in academic surgery. These qualities give department chairs and program directors confidence in an applicant's potential to help define the character of their residency program, which is left behind as part of their professional and academic legacies.

18.3   Interviewing with Other Faculty Members

Although non-administrative faculty members may not be directly responsible for the overall culture of a residency program, these surgeons play an important role in forming an impression of residency applicants during the interview process. Faculty surgeons are aware of the goals and priorities of the department chair and program director for the residents that comprise the program. An applicant's story of their passion and career vision adds validation to the impressions formed by the chair and program director when integrated with the responses to other faculty member interviews.

Non-administrative faculty members may not directly ask questions of an applicant's future impact on surgery. Nonetheless, weaving the story of how an applicant envisions their career advancing surgical practice is an effective way to convey professional values and ambition in addition to leadership potential.

18.4   Interacting/Interviewing with Residents

A residency is viewed as "family" by the residents; they care deeply about who matches in their program. The passion and ambition that can set applicants apart during interviews with faculty and leadership must be addressed differently when interacting with residents, even at academic surgery programs. While individual residents may be interested in learning about your professional goals and aspirations, most residents seek to evaluate applicants based on their affability, integrity, and ability to interact with others on a team. While residents may care about applicants' career ambitions, it is less important for applicants to convey their academic passions to residents than to faculty surgeons.

If a resident asks an applicant about their specific interests in academic surgery, the applicant should feel free to communicate their ideas as they feel is appropriate. However, applicants do not need to weave their professional story into conversations with residents as they might with faculty surgeons during interviews.

18.5 Summary

These insights will help applicants interviewing at academic surgery residency programs to communicate a strong, persuasive case for *why* and *how* they will become valuable residents and future leaders in surgery. There are many interviewing skills critical to performing well in interviews that are not discussed here. Applicants would be wise to prepare for interviews in a well-rounded manner. This chapter highlights specific priorities of academic surgery programs that may assist applicants who desire to distinguish themselves during interviews at highly regarded surgery residency programs. Once applicants are granted an interview, they have a unique opportunity to sell themselves and convince residency programs that they deserve to train to become the future leaders in surgery.

Chapter 19
I Am a Surgery Resident Now, 10 Things I Wish I Had Learned as a Medical Student

Jared R. Gallaher and Laura N. Purcell

Abstract The transition from medical school to residency is a period of significant adjustment. The goal of this chapter is to highlight several areas that are critical to pay attention to during this time and plan for in advance of beginning training. These are ten of the most important lessons we wish we had learned as medical students prior to surgical residency although all of these apply to other specialties. This is taken from personal perspective as well as input from peers and the medical literature. We hope this list facilitates personal reflection on how you can learn from our experiences and begin the process of working towards your own professional development.

The transition from medical school to residency is a period of significant adjustment. The goal of this chapter is to highlight several areas that are critical to pay attention to during this time and plan for in advance of beginning training. These are ten of the most important lessons we wish we had learned as medical students prior to surgical residency although all of these apply to other specialties. This is taken from personal perspective as well as input from peers and the medical literature. We hope this list facilitates personal reflection on how you can learn from our experiences and begin the process of working towards your own professional development.

19.1 Develop Organizational Skills Now

Years of schooling have taught you the fundamental skills needed to keep your school work organized. However residency will challenge your capacity to organize your work, as well as your personal life. This is illustrated in a recent study showing

J.R. Gallaher, MD, MPH (✉) • L.N. Purcell
University of North Carolina, Chapel Hill, NC, USA
e-mail: jared.gallaher@unchealth.unc.edu; Laura.Purcell@unchealth.unc.edu

© Springer International Publishing Switzerland 2017
M.J. Englesbe, M.O. Meyers (eds.), *A How To Guide For Medical Students*,
Success in Academic Surgery, DOI 10.1007/978-3-319-42897-0_19

that residency program directors identified poor organizational skills as a primary concern for incoming interns (Lyss-Lerman et al. 2009). Medical school is the perfect time to focus on improving your organizational skills. We suggest focusing on these three areas.

During your clinical rotations experiment with different systems of organizing patient information and tasks. As a third-year medical student you will likely handle up to five patients on most services, but as an intern you may be managing as many as thirty patients. Medical school is a great time to practice different approaches to organizing information in order to find what works best for you; some of the best techniques can be learned from strong residents with whom you are working. Many of your responsibilities as a resident will be administrative, either in implementing plans or organizing data for complex patients. Consequently, it is impossible to succeed as an intern without a foundational set of organizational skills.

Second, you will need to balance clinical work responsibilities with other non-clinical expectations. This includes activities like research, board certification, loan repayment, and medical student education. Your department will fill your inbox with emails that need timely responses. You will also need to keep track of your medical license and when you are participating in research: communications from your IRB, abstract, conference, and funding deadlines.

Lastly, as you have already experienced during medical school, your personal life does not stop during training despite the increased level of responsibility. Bills still need to be paid and that pile of laundry will not wash itself. Experiment with different systems that help you keep track of day to day life like automatic bill pay. There are also many mobile apps useful for this purpose that can keep important aspect of your life in order, such as your parents' birthdays.

While medical school is very challenging, your last years of medical school and your residency training will add additional layers of complexity and a substantial amount of new data for you to organize and utilize. Establish these good habits now.

19.2   Work Well with Others

During school it is easy to focus on individual performance and overlook that healthcare is fundamentally a team sport. The delivery of quality care requires an incredible number of people working in synchrony. The healthcare team extends out from fellow residents and attendings to the mid-level providers, pharmacists, nurses, case managers, and hospital staff that make the hospital function. It is critical to develop strong collaboration skills as quality teamwork improves patient outcomes and also helps you reach your goals – a patient's safe discharge.

The importance of teamwork in clinical care is a point of emphasis in health services research. A recently published systematic review showed that effective teamwork correlated with positive patient outcomes (McKinley 2016). There is also evidence that programs like interdisciplinary rounds only improve clinical outcomes if they increase teamwork (O'Leary et al. 2016). Effective teamwork requires robust communication, task coordination, and strong leadership.

As a physician in training, you will have a natural leadership position on the team. Take this role seriously by establishing patterns of healthy team interaction. The Golden Rule, "Do to others as you would have them do to you" applies aptly in teamwork development. Treat others well and it will usually be reciprocated. As your training progresses, your confidence will grow but you must guard against arrogance. Seek humility by receiving feedback well and be constructive with advice to others. In addition to helping patients, other members of the health care team will be critical for your professional development through personal support, constructive criticism, and task-sharing for common goals.

In the midst of stress and exhaustion, working well with others is challenging. However, it is these moments where you need your coworkers most to provide excellent care to your patients and to help you grow as a physician.

19.3   Establish Habits of Personal Responsibility

One of the most convenient, but most damaging, attitudes to develop in medical school is the avoidance of responsibility for patient care. During your third and fourth year of medical school you will follow patients, present their clinical course during rounds, and even perform their procedures. However, you will be aware that the resident (and by extension the attending) is ultimately responsible for placing their orders for the day, writing their progress note, and supervising your involvement. When you are busy, exhausted, stressed, or simply have other plans, it will be easy to think of this safety net as excusing you from responsibility.

Working long, stressful hours is challenging in any profession. Medicine is unique in that nearly every decision you make has a potential harmful effect on another person. Taking care of patients is a special responsibility that demands a significant professional commitment. As a medical student, you are protected by the residents and faculty working over you. When you start residency this changes. Consequently, medical school is a great time to start developing two habits that will make it easier for you to take responsibility for your patients as a resident.

First, avoid signing out tasks or studies to follow-up at night for your patients. As a medical student, your time is often protected allowing you to go home before the work is done. Discern when it is appropriate to leave and when it might be better for your learning to stay later to see a procedure on one of your patients or follow the course of someone critically ill. If staying at the hospital is not practical, practice following-up on your patients from home.

Second, challenge yourself to know more about your patients than anyone else. The harder you work to follow-up investigations, find outside records, and obtain a more thorough history, the more responsible you will feel for you patients and their outcome. As a student, your role as a conduit of patient information for the team is invaluable and will help you develop healthy habits useful for the rest of your career.

Take your personal responsibility for your patients seriously now. Habits you build as a student will build a foundation that lasts a career.

19.4 Find Good Mentors

All of us know less than we realize. Thankfully, mentors with experience and expertise help guide us through decisions and our professional development. As a medical student, you should start seeking out mentors and the earlier, the better. They may be basic science instructors, small group leaders, your anatomy lab teacher, an attending you worked with, or a resident you connected with on a clinical rotation. All of these people are well ahead in the training process and can help you with decisions and give you advice in challenging circumstances.

One of the first major decisions you will make in medical school is your clinical specialty. Mentors often play a significant role in this process either by helping you discern a good personal fit or by serving as a role model in a particular specialty (Thakur et al. 2001). During The Match, you will seek guidance on programs to apply to and how to order your rank list. Your mentors may offer important perspectives when selecting a program, write letters of recommendation, make calls to program directors, and network on your behalf (Mayer et al. 2001).

Outside of career decisions, mentors are vital for your professional development. This includes providing feedback on your clinical performance and teamwork effectiveness. It also involves teaching you basic skills in non-clinical areas such as research. Your first mentors may be your first co-authors on a research project or direct you to the right journal for a paper you write.

However, finding the right mentor requires initiative. Most of these people are very busy, just like you. You should seek out potential mentors by scheduling a time to meet and expressing your desire for a mentor relationship. Some medical schools or residency programs may have formalized programs but evidence in some specialties suggests this is an unmet need and you should you not rely on others to establish these relationships for you (Dhami et al. 2016).

19.5 Learn Work-Life Balance Early

Physician burnout and work-life balance are buzzwords in medical education. As future residents, these topics will be featured during many meetings and grand rounds. Burnout is defined as emotional exhaustion, depersonalization, and feelings of reduced personal accomplishment. Across all specialties, reported burnout rates average 50 %. These feelings are not limited to residency; medical student burnout is reported as high as 45 % (Ishak et al. 2009).

Do not have the false impression that once you reach residency and the 80-h work week that there will be much time outside of work. Unfortunately there is not. In residency, much like medical school, there is always something more you could be doing: studying for tomorrow's operating room cases, working on a research project, or finishing clinic notes.

When applying to medical schools and residency programs we are pushed to become modern Renaissance men and women. Our applications are full of academic, art, and athletic achievements with long lists of hobbies to prove we are well rounded. You will be unable to sustain all your hobbies and extracurricular activities during residency. Instead, identify the aspects of your life most important to you. What rejuvenates you? Whether it is friends, family, faith, running, reading, painting, or playing the trumpet, maintaining these pieces of your life will make you more resilient, a better doctor, and keep your life a little more "normal."

19.6 Residency Is a Journey

The vast amount of medical knowledge is exponentially expanding. In 1950, the doubling time of medical knowledge was about 50 years; in the 1980s, 7 years; and in 2010, it was estimated to be about 3.5 years. By 2020, the doubling rate of medical knowledge is expected to be 0.2 years, a mere 73 days (Densen 2011).

"He who would learn to fly 1 day must first learn to stand and walk and run and climb and dance; one cannot fly into flying." Nietzsche's quote is applicable to becoming a doctor and starting residency. You will not be expected to know everything about medicine and general surgery or function independently on July 1st. On day one, you will be a step ahead if you can find the bathroom and have a functioning EMR password.

A surgery residency is structured as a tiered, 5-year program for a reason. The hospital is structured for patient safety and your education. At no point will you be alone in the hospital caring for patients, even on night call. There are nurses with significantly more experience than you, upper level general surgery residents, and cardiology fellows. No matter how many times you read *Dublin's Rapid Interpretation of EKG* before starting residency, you will not be expected to get a patient suffering from a myocardial infarction to the cardiac catheterization laboratory independently.

Over the course of the 5-year general surgery residency, you will gain the knowledge and skills needed to become an independent practicing surgeon. Start developing those needed skills in medical school. Prepare for cases by reading about the patient prior to stepping in the operating room. Understand the indications for each procedure, the anatomy for that specific operation, and complications of each surgical procedure before scrubbing for the case, and meet the patients prior to the operation. These people are putting their trust in your surgical team at a vulnerable time in their lives and should respect their trust. The energy invested is directly related to the knowledge and experience gained. At the end of your residency it will be your operating room, so start practicing the skills now!

19.7 Delve into Research

As an academic surgeon, research in some form or another will be a constant aspect of your life. There is exciting and important research being done at all medical schools in many fields, including: basic science, clinical, translational, and outcomes-based research. Get involved! Many professors will have projects underway and more often than not, they will need and want assistance. Find a surgeon you would like to work with and ask if they have a project. The worst that can happen is they say "No."

The benefits to participating in research are twofold. Research experience will narrow your program search and strengthen your application. Finding research you love has the ability to focus your residency program search to institutions that excel in the research that excites you. If you find research is not part of your future, it will steer you away from academic programs.

In addition, involvement in surgical research may strengthen a residency application and set applications apart in a competitive general surgery applicant pool. In a study surveying general surgery program directors involvement in clinical and basic science research was an important secondary criterion for potential surgery residents with directors (Melendez et al. 2008). Through research you can obtain a more powerful letter of recommendation by establishing a strong relationship with a professor, produce tangible evidence for interest in surgery, and provide important talking points within a residency interview.

19.8 Explore Your Interests

"Twenty years from now you will be more disappointed by the things that you didn't do than by the ones you did do. So throw off the bowlines. Sail away from the safe harbor. Catch the trade winds in your sails. Explore. Dream. Discover." This popular quote attributed to Mark Twain, describes the exploration one should pursue in medical school. Medical school is unable to teach or give exposure to all areas of a rapidly growing medical field. If a field peaks your interest, take the opportunity to explore that area.

Seek a diversity of experiences during medical school. Use your elective months in third and fourth year to explore medical fields outside of surgery. This might include radiology to understand how to read imaging, anesthesiology to explore what happens on the other side of the curtain in the operating room, pathology to follow the specimens surgeons remove, or whatever strikes your fancy. Another opportunity are global health experiences. Medical students who have undertaken international experiences have more confidence in their diagnostic skills, a greater understanding of the importance of public health, increased respect of cross-cultural communication and competency, and appreciate health care allocation and costs (Thompson et al. 2003; Drain et al. 2007).

During fourth year, we recommend pursuing away rotations at different academic institutions. As you are applying for residencies and creating your program match list, these experiences provide a framework for evaluating your needs and desires from a residency program. Perhaps most importantly, these experiences help identify what you do not want in a future career or specific residency.

19.9   Cultivate a Healthy Perspective

Perhaps one of the more challenging aspects of your medical education is keeping a healthy perspective on your work and training. Many medical students enter their training idealistic about patient care and the altruism of practicing medicine. These feelings may unfortunately fade as long hours and stress build up. It is important to cultivate a healthy perspective on your work through some simple practices.

First, accept that you will make mistakes. Perfectionism may have helped you excel in school, but in clinical practice much of your learning happens on the job. You will not be prepared for your first day of your internship but you will learn quickly with the help of others and through your mistakes. Challenge yourself to use errors as motivators to work harder, care more, and utilize the help offered to you by your team. When you make a mistake, talk to someone on your team or a co-resident. Research has shown that regular team discussions help prevent burnout among surgery residents (Chaput et al. 2015).

Second, express daily appreciation to your teachers and co-workers for their contribution to your education. Gratitude will center your perspective as a constant reminder that you depend on others for your professional development.

Lastly, continue to invest time in the volunteer activities. This is admittedly challenging given the time commitment of medical school and residency but will help you maintain a perspective on why you pursued a career in medicine. Interest in global health has been growing in recent years but there are many local volunteer opportunities as well. Finding a way to incorporate this into your life will grow your appreciation for your job.

In the end, you are training to be a physician in order to help others. Seek our practices that help cultivate a perspective that acknowledges you are fallible, that you depend on others, and that acts of service are the driving force behind your work.

19.10   Attitude Is Everything

It is no secret that residency can be challenging and immensely frustrating at times. Balancing the demands of attendings, patients, and nurses with clinical and research responsibilities, while also trying to maintain a work-life balance is incredibly stressful.

We challenge you to keep a positive attitude. Finish medical school and start residency by setting the right tone personally. The path to becoming a physician and surgeon is an incredible journey so relish in the experience. This being said, there are days where a vent session will be therapeutic and necessary.

Maintaining a positive attitude throughout the process can be challenging, but it will make you a better team player and has shown to improve your mental health. Scheier et al. describe three ways a positive attitude can improve an individual's ability to cope with stress, which are as follows:

1. *"Breathe"* – provides break from managing the stress
2. *"Sustain"* – bolster perseverance and drive when times become most difficult
3. *"Restore"* – improving ability to recover from stress by restoring diminished resources (Scheier and Carver 1985)

These three characteristics will aid your resiliency and make your residency experience more enjoyable and fulfilling.

In "Invictus" William Earnest Henley wrote, "I am the master of my fate: I am the captain of my soul." You have the opportunity to direct your medical school and residency journey. By doing so with a positive outlook and learning from our experiences, you will be successful in any residency you choose.

References

Chaput B, Bertheuil N, Jacques J, Smilevitch D, Bekara F, Soler P, et al. Professional burnout among plastic surgery residents: can it be prevented? Outcomes of a national survey. Ann Plast Surg. 2015;75(1):2–8.

Densen P. Challenges and opportunities facing medical education. Trans Am Clin Climatol Assoc. 2011;122:48–58.

Dhami G, Gao W, Gensheimer MF, Trister AD, Kane G, Zeng J. Mentorship programs in radiation oncology residency training programs: a critical unmet need. Int J Radiat Oncol Biol Phys. 2016;94(1):27–30.

Drain PK, Primack A, Hunt DD, Fawzi WW, Holmes KK, Gardner P. Global health in medical education: a call for more training and opportunities. Acad Med. 2007;82(3):226–30.

Ishak WW, Lederer S, Mandili C, Nikravesh R, Seligman L, Vasa M, et al. Burnout during residency training: a literature review. J Grad Med Educ. 2009;1(2):236–42.

Lyss-Lerman P, Teherani A, Aagaard E, Loeser H, Cooke M, Harper GM. What training is needed in the fourth year of medical school? Views of residency program directors. Acad Med. 2009;84(7):823–9.

Mayer KL, Perez RV, Ho HS. Factors affecting choice of surgical residency training program. J Surg Res. 2001;98(2):71–5.

McKinley DW. Evaluating team performance: a systematic review. In: Assessing competence in professional performance across disciplines and professions. Switzerland: Springer; 2016. p. 285–329.

Melendez MM, Xu X, Sexton TR, Shapiro MJ, Mohan EP. The importance of basic science and clinical research as a selection criterion for general surgery residency programs. J Surg Educ. 2008;65(2):151–4.

O'Leary KJ, Johnson JK, Auerbach AD. Do interdisciplinary rounds improve patient outcomes? Only if they improve teamwork. J Hosp Med. 2016;11(7):524–5.

Scheier MF, Carver CS. Optimism, coping, and health: assessment and implications of generalized outcome expectancies. Health Psychol. 1985;4(3):219–47.

Thakur A, Fedorka P, Ko C, Buchmiller-Crair TL, Atkinson JB, Fonkalsrud EW. Impact of mentor guidance in surgical career selection. J Pediatr Surg. 2001;36(12):1802–4.

Thompson MJ, Huntington MK, Hunt DD, Pinsky LE, Brodie JJ. Educational effects of international health electives on U.S. and Canadian medical students and residents: a literature review. Acad Med. 2003;78(3):342–7.

Chapter 20
Case Study: Foundations of a Successful Academic Surgery Development Program

Alyssa Mazurek, David Cron, Charles Hwang, Stephanie DeBolle, Rishindra M. Reddy, and Jason Pradarelli

Abstract Medical students are often searching for ways to demonstrate leadership and to engage their peers in the career development process. At the University of Michigan Medical School, an academic surgery development program was created with the goal of providing opportunities to tackle these challenging aspects of professional development. This chapter provides an example of how medical students, residents, and faculty collaborated to facilitate productive relationships between medical students and surgeons. Many elements of Michigan's "SCRUBS" group outlined below can be replicated or modified at any medical school. For those who see benefit and utility in the programming outlined here, we encourage medical students to take the initiative and reach out to faculty members, mentors and peers. Current medical students can be leaders at their own institutions by establishing career exposure and development, which will in turn benefit the futures of many other medical students.

Medical students are often searching for ways to demonstrate leadership and to engage their peers in the career development process. At the University of Michigan Medical School, an academic surgery development program was created with the goal of providing opportunities to tackle these challenging aspects of professional development. This chapter provides an example of how medical students, residents, and faculty collaborated to facilitate productive relationships between medical students and surgeons. Many elements of Michigan's "SCRUBS" group outlined

A. Mazurek (✉) • D. Cron • C. Hwang • S. DeBolle • R.M. Reddy
University of Michigan, Ann Arbor, MI, USA
e-mail: mazureka@med.umich.edu; dcron@med.umich.edu; umichuck@med.umich.edu; sdebolle@med.umich.edu; reddyrm@med.umich.edu

J. Pradarelli
Brigham and Women's Hospital, Boston, MA, USA
e-mail: jcprad@med.umish.edu

below can be replicated or modified at any medical school. For those who see benefit and utility in the programming outlined here, we encourage medical students to take the initiative and reach out to faculty members, mentors and peers. Current medical students can be leaders at their own institutions by establishing career exposure and development, which will in turn benefit the futures of many other medical students.

20.1 Background

While accredited medical institutions provide reasonable exposure to core specialties through clinical clerkships, it is impossible to provide exposure to all medical subspecialties. Thus, for those potentially interested in surgery or other procedural specialties, early exposure to and mentorship via extracurricular activities can help students make informed career decisions. Early preparation will equip students with the tools to be strong applicants for competitive residencies. This was the goal of the original SCRUBS program, founded by Dr. Mark B. Orringer from the University of Michigan. SCRUBS is the surgery interest group at the University of Michigan Medical School that facilitates exposure to surgery in order to recruit and develop the future leaders in academic surgery. The program began in 2002, as a commitment to cultivating interest and exposure for pre-clinical and clinical medical students. Since then, the group has developed into a broader program that supports mentorship, research, clinical skills development, and career guidance. SCRUBS is organized into:

- Networking and outreach
- Clinical competency
- Research

Each branch coordinates activities to help facilitate leadership development and involvement for students interested in surgery and other procedural subspecialties.

Ultimately, SCRUBS aims to form a meaningful link between students and the invaluable resource of surgery faculty and residents. SCRUBS provides opportunities for students of varying interest levels. Informal conversations with faculty surgeons provide an introduction to surgery for pre-clinical students with fledgling interest. More committed students can pursue surgical research opportunities and begin to develop technical surgical skills in preparation for their surgical clerkship.

20.2 Networking & Outreach

Is surgery the right fit for me? Many pre-clinical students experience anxiety over the idea of choosing a specialty, and many have no prior exposure to surgery. The outreach component of SCRUBS provides a venue for students to explore and ask questions regarding a surgical career and lifestyle. SCRUBS capitalizes on the availability of experienced medical students, residents, and faculty in order to provide pre-clinical students with a realistic perception of the training and lifestyle encompassed within surgery. SCRUBS organizes monthly lunch or dinner talks, where faculty with diverse backgrounds and experiences discuss their paths, career decisions and lifestyle. These began as dinners graciously hosted by Dr. Orringer at his home. These evenings included faculty presentations followed by instruction on basic surgical skills. The intimate nature and opportunity to interact with surgeons from all walks of life in a personal setting made the "Orringer Dinners" a favorite SCRUBS event. These dinners have since evolved to rotate at a different faculty member's house each month. With the faculty member opening up their home to medical students, they truly open the door into a personal side of surgery that may be difficult to emulate in any other way.

How do I find a good mentor amongst the many faculty present at an institution? Once one is identified, how do I build a meaningful and productive relationship? SCRUBS aims to connect pre-clinical medical students with clinical medical students, residents, and faculty. Each year, SCRUBS reaches out to surgical faculty members and inquires whether they are willing to act as mentors to students. Once this list is compiled, it is sent out to SCRUBS students as a resource to guide their initial exploration of mentors who may have similar interests or desired career paths. The faculty members involved in SCRUBS are extremely dedicated to helping medical students succeed. They will meet with students and point them in the right direction for finding a professional or research mentor. In addition, the variety of SCRUBS activities facilitate the building of relationships between the students and faculty and residents.

So I want to be a surgeon, what next? Many of the students involved in SCRUBS have a strong interest in surgery, and given the competitive nature of the field, desire ways in which they can excel during clinical clerkships and residency interviews. SCRUBS hosts several M4 panels and mixers in order to connect pre-clinical medical students with upperclassmen who have successfully gone through the process of applying and matching into a surgery residency. The guidance offered by M4s is invaluable, as they have just gone through many of the experiences about which underclassmen seek advice. Events with the M4s provide an opportunity for pre-clinical students to learn how to succeed during clinical clerkships and how to best prepare for and apply to surgery residency. In addition, these conversations often further ignite pre-clinical students' interest in the field. Once a student's interest in surgery is generated, SCRUBS offers a variety of other programming to jumpstart their career development.

20.3　Cultivating Clinical Competency

What does the technical side of surgery entail, and will I be any good at it?　These are common concerns raised by many students interested in surgery. The clinical component of SCRUBS provides students with a preview into the technical skills, work environment and teaching elements of a career in academic surgery. SCRUBS provides many opportunities for students to do basic surgical skills as well as in-depth practice for interested students. Students gain early exposure to foundational surgical skills through events facilitated by surgical faculty and residents in the Clinical Simulation Center. These sessions provide an intimate setting for students to learn skills in suturing, knot tying, and laparoscopy. Sessions also cover critical care skills, such as intubation and central line placement that are relevant in many areas of medicine. With avid participation in these sessions, students gain comfort with technical skills that will help them shine during their clinical clerkships.

What should I do in the clinic or operating room to avoid causing trouble or being in the way? How do I productively contribute to patient care?　Students learn to navigate professional environments through "Introduction to the OR" sessions where faculty discuss appropriate behavior and actions to take while shadowing and assisting in the operating room. These sessions are consistently cited as the first time pre-clinical medical students learn to scrub, which often launch future prospects to scrub in with their mentors and experience educational cases. As reiterated by many of the surgical faculty, one of the key elements to a medical student doing well in their surgery clerkship is possessing "situational awareness," and understanding how they can contribute to patient care. Sessions such as "Intro to the OR" provide a safe space for students to begin developing, and subsequently, practicing these skills.

What can leadership look like?　Surgical residency programs across the country desire students who will become leaders and who embrace the opportunity to teach their peers. Based on the ever-growing emphasis on leadership in medical education, the clinical component of SCRUBS also entails a Teaching Fellowship program that provides a structure for students to experience leadership akin to what physicians in academic medicine practice. The premise of the program involves fourth year medical students (M4s) teaching second year medical students (M2s) who then teach first year medical students (M1s), benefitting both pre-clinical and clinical medical students simultaneously. M4s hone their teaching skills, while M2s reinforce their foundational knot tying and suturing skills. Upon successful completion of a predetermined list of requirements and demonstrated competencies, M2s then lead small group sessions targeted to M1s. This program has received very positive feedback from all levels of student involvement, promoted interclass collaboration, and has allowed expansion of SCRUBS activities that were previously limited by resident and faculty availability.

20.4   Building Your Research Repertoire

How do I find a research mentor and engage in publishable research while in medical school? Many of the medical students applying into surgical residency programs have extensive research experience and publications. However, pre-clinical medical students often find it difficult to navigate the lengthy lists of surgical faculty and residents when searching for potential research mentors. To address this concern, SCRUBS developed a research branch that is devoted to helping connect pre-clinical medical students with research mentors that both align with the students' interests and offer a productive experience. The SCRUBS Surgery Olympics is an example of one such program. This program commences during the summer after the M1 year and continues throughout the M2 year. "Olympic" teams consist of one surgery faculty mentor and 4–5 students. Students are tasked with completing a clinical research project, writing and presenting an abstract, and writing a manuscript. The main goal is to foster communication skills – teaching students how to present findings in tables and figures and write clear and concise clinical research manuscripts. The Olympics program also includes a technical component. For this part of the program, teams of students practice knot tying and suturing, both in structured sessions held by residents and with one-on-one coaching by their faculty mentor. This program culminates in a competition in which teams battle head to head in technical skills, followed by oral presentations given at a Department of Surgery Grand Rounds where faculty members score abstracts and presentations. This SCRUBS Surgery Olympics program offers a more time-intensive exposure to the field of academic surgery and has received phenomenal feedback from both students and faculty.

20.5   Taking Hold of the Future

SCRUBS is a student-run group that serves students and provides opportunities. It would not be possible without the unwavering support and dedication from faculty, residents and the medical student leaders. This program provides a head start on preparing for clinical clerkship, as well as opportunities to interact with experienced residents and faculty who provide advice and guidance. The more students know, the better prepared they are. Ultimately, the goal of SCRUBS is to inspire students to become leaders in their field and present themselves as mature residency applicants.

Programs such as SCRUBS offer extraordinary learning outside the classroom. Medical students should actively seek out programs while in medical school that offer a place for leadership development, early career exposure, and access to residents and faculty. If one does not already exist, students can work to create something new that will connect the medical school to the residents and faculty in a novel way. The power behind this program lies in the connections and the invaluable resources generated for medical students. By establishing strong relationships with mentors, having a diverse collection of experiences and making informed career decisions, medical students can take an active role in creating a successful and bright future.

Index

© Springer International Publishing Switzerland 2017
M.J. Englesbe, M.O. Meyers (eds.), *A How To Guide For Medical Students*,
Success in Academic Surgery, DOI 10.1007/978-3-319-42897-0

Printed in the United States
By Bookmasters